Stress Incontinence Explained

Male and female incontinence

Urinary incontinence treatment, bladder problems, overactive bladder, urge incontinence, incontinence products, all covered

Published by Cleal Publishing

Copyright ©2016 Cleal Publishing

ISBN (978-0-9955610-1-4)

Disclaimer

While the author and publisher have made all available efforts to ensure the information contained in this book was correct at press time, neither the author nor publisher assumes and hereby disclaims any liability to any party for damages, disruption, or loss caused by the use and application, directly or indirectly, of any information presented including any errors. This book is not meant to substitute for medical advice from a qualified healthcare professional. The reader should regularly consult with a healthcare professional in matters relating to his/her health, particularly with respect to any of the symptoms discussed that may require professional treatment.

The accuracy and completeness of information provided herein and opinions stated herein are not guaranteed or warranted to produce any particular results, and the advice and strategies contained herein may not be suitable for every individual.

Contents

INTRODUCTION

Man is not a machine
that can be remodelled for quite other purposes
as occasion demands,
in the hope that it will go on functioning
as regularly as before
but in a quite different way.
He carries his whole history with him;
in his very structure
is written the history of mankind.

Carl Gustav Jung

Stress incontinence? What is that? It is the involuntary, spontaneous leakage of urine, a condition that most likely affects your work and personal life, right? Is it a part of the normal process of aging? No. Is it treatable? Yes, but you need to find strength and motivation in order to tackle this issue. This book is designed to help you understand why it has happened to you or someone you know, or simply to find out what is it and how you can take your health into your own hands. Can it be prevented? There are a few measures you can take, such as doing some exercises, eating healthier, drinking the recommended amount of fluids, and reducing the use of cigarettes and alcohol. You will read about how this problem is diagnosed and treated.

Don't give up hope, because you can do it. This book will show you how to manage this condition.

1.   Anatomy and structure of urinary system.

Little processes constantly take place in our bodies; something is built, while something else is destroyed. Busy cells work with electrolytes and enzymes and change one type of chemical to another type to create energy.

These processes require a system that removes all of the resulting waste products from the body. Water, electrolytes, toxins, products of medicines, and body chemicals go through the bloodstream to our kidneys, where they are filtered into urine and secreted.

Our urinary system consists of kidneys, the ureters, the urinary bladder, and the urethra. Each of the two kidneys is fed by blood vessels that bring blood to be filtered. Through a long path of tubelets in the kidneys, 99% of the content is reabsorbed into the bloodstream. Why? So we don't lose precious water and electrolytes that are crucial for our functioning. Then, the urine leaves the kidney and flows through the ureters into the urinary bladder. The wall of the urinary bladder is elastic, allowing it to fill to a certain volume, and has a smooth detrusor muscle that can endure even the biggest pressures and is responsible for complete emptying of the bladder. As the bladder is filled more and more, and the pressure in it rises, pressure on the sphincter, the part of the urethra that acts like a door, also increases. That sends out impulses through the spinal cord to the brain, which in turn sends impulses that give us a strong need to empty the bladder, or urinate. If the urination doesn't happen, the pressure lowers for a little while, allowing us to postpone urination. After a certain amount of time, pressure rises again, creating a stronger need to empty the bladder. This can occur a couple of times, until the pressure on the sphincter is larger than the pressure it can take, and urination happens. In a healthy individual, this urination is voluntarily controlled, but it is involuntary if some part of the urinary system isn't functioning the way it is supposed to. This couldn't happen in a healthy urinary system, not even with growing intra-abdominal pressure, as happens when we cough, laugh, sneeze, lift heavy things, etc. [1]

The urethra of a man is much longer (average length 20cm) than the female urethra (average length 3cm). There are two sphincters: the one at the transition between the bladder and urethra is called the internal sphincter and is a distal part of the detrusor muscle. The external sphincter is located in the inner third of the urethra or, in males, in the area inferior to the prostate. The inner sphincter is made of smooth muscles and therefore we can't have voluntary control over it. The external is made out of striated muscles, which we can voluntarily control.

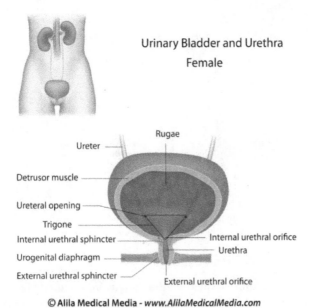

Figure 1 Position of kidneys, ureters, bladder, and urethra in a woman's body. The bladder is shown with its muscle layer and trigonum where, in two upper points, ureters enter the bladder, and the point below, where the urethra begins.

The outer part of the urethra is surrounded by the strong muscles of pelvic floor. If you imagine that all of the abdominal pressure is supported from the lower side, with only the muscles around the urethra and rectum, you can see that those muscles must be very strong to keep the organs from dropping farther down. They act like a hammock holding the organs and other structures. There is also a group of muscles called the pelvic diaphragm. Four muscles are involved: the pubococcygeus, iliococcygeus, ischiococcygeus, and coccygeus. The muscles are attached to pelvic bones and they form the levator ani muscle. This muscle has three openings: one for the rectum, one for the urethra, and, in females, an opening for the vagina. There is also connective tissue that supports this complex. The most important ligaments are the urethropelvic ligament, pubocervical fascia, cardinal ligaments, and uterosacral ligaments. If any of them is damaged, that would cause prolapse in the organs of the pelvis and dysfunction in holding the urine. [2]

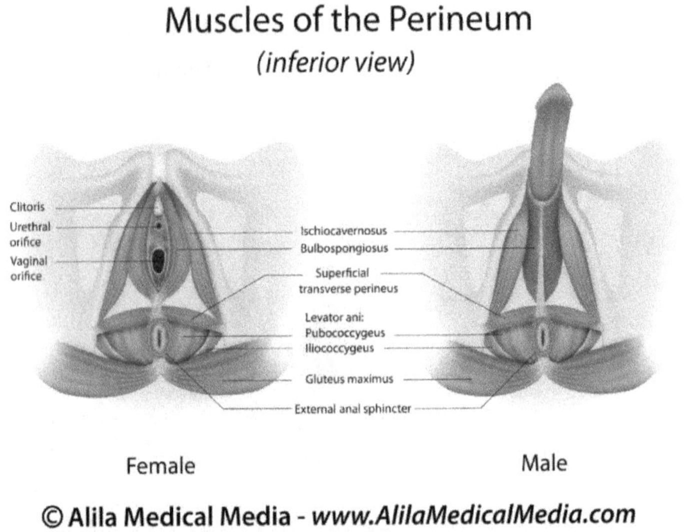

Muscles of the Perineum
(inferior view)

Clitoris
Urethral orifice
Vaginal orifice

Ischiocavernosus
Bulbospongiosus
Superficial transverse perineus
Levator ani:
Pubococcygeus
Iliococcygeus
Gluteus maximus
External anal sphincter

Female   Male

© Alila Medical Media - www.AlilaMedicalMedia.com

Figure 2 Muscles of perineum in women (left) and men(right). Levator ani muscle consists of pubococcygeus, iliococcygeus, ischiococcygeus and coccygeus muscles.

1.1 Differences in male and female anatomy of genitourinary system

Male and female development is determined early in the process of fetal development, and is influenced by the possession or lack of the Y chromosome. Female-determined genes are carried by two X chromosomes, creating a XX pair of sex chromosomes, while in men there are X and Y chromosomes. The Y chromosome is much smaller than the X chromosome, but it holds the genetic information about the development and growth of male gonads and sex organs. [3]

The male urinary system is conjoined with the reproductive tract. The reproductive tract consists of the testicles, the epididymis, and the vas deferens, which then leads to the urethra. The urinary and reproductive systems are joined in the urethra. The urethra is approximately 20cm long; it goes from the urinary bladder through the prostate and on to the external opening in the genitals.

The male urethra is less likely to be affected by external factors such as bacteria because the bacteria need to pass a longer distance before they reach the bladder. On the other hand, the prostate endangers the urine flow if it is enlarged and therefore makes the bladder retain the urine, which could be a favourable condition in the case of infections, but can also cause incontinence.

The female urinary system goes from the kidneys through the ureters to the urinary bladder; from there, the urine passes through the urethra. The urethra is 3-4cm long and is prone to infections. There is some speculation about whether the female bladder is smaller than the male's. The answer lies in differences of general body physique. People who are taller or bigger in mass and height have bigger bladders and vice versa.

Reasons that incontinence occurs more in women is are the shortness of the urethra and the weakening of pelvic floor muscles that takes place, especially after childbirth and with aging. [4]

2. What is incontinence?

When the urine is involuntarily let out of the bladder, it is called urinary incontinence. Some complain of urine leaking spontaneously, and some that urine leaks when they cough, laugh, or work out. This can be connected to the dysfunction of the bladder itself, neural dysfunction, or damage to or weakening of the pelvic diaphragm. Incontinence is involved with loss of urine without any symptoms, such as pain, tenderness, or itching. It can happen any time during daylight activities, which is, obviously, uncomfortable.

2.1 How many people have trouble with incontinence? Epidemiology of incontinence.

Urinary incontinence brings with it failure to function successfully in the work place, with colleagues and friends, and even with family. The condition is often kept a secret. The person at first ignores the problem, until a couple of months and even years pass, and then it really starts to have effects on his or her psychological sphere. It is usually undiagnosed for approximately 6-9 years, since people are ashamed to admit to a physician and even to their family that the problem exists. They usually think that confessing the problem will mark them as unworthy to be around. It affects between 50 and 84% of the population in elderly institutions. Between 50 and 70 % of women don't seek medical attention because of the fear of social rejection.

In the U.S., between 10 and 13 million people suffer from this condition and there are more than 200 million people in the world with this condition, which makes it a serious problem that affects 35% of population.

It is twice as common in women as in men. Women are more vulnerable after vaginal baby delivery and after some surgeries. It is understandable that it occurs more frequently with elderly people since the generalizing atrophy and weakening of muscles develop with time all over the body. It can also affect children older than the age of 5 (7%) and 10% to 35% of adults are affected. [5]

2.2 Types of incontinence

As previously mentioned, incontinence can be caused by many factors as the consequences of childbirth, aging, and other medical conditions. Therefore, there are several types of incontinence:

- Stress incontinence
- Urge incontinence
- Overflow incontinence
- Functional incontinence
- Mixed incontinence
- Transient incontinence

2.2.1. Stress incontinence

Stress incontinence is a condition caused by several factors, of which older age and female sex are the most important. The urine is involuntarily "escaping" when a person laughs, coughs, lifts heavy objects, sneezes, exerts, or runs. With such activities, intra-abdominal pressure increases on the bladder and the muscles of pelvic floor, which, if they are weakened, or if the bladder-urethra junction isn't at the right angle and the bladder neck is without support, taken together cause the loss of control over the urine flow, and it leaks out of the bladder. A person at the beginning usually uses pads, on average 1-3 a day. This is when incontinence is mild. Leakages don't usually happen at night. The incontinence is considered severe when a person leaks large amounts of urine and has to change pads very frequently. In this case, it is more important to consult the health care provider, because some serious conditions can develop, such as fistulas when bladder and urethra are connected through another canal without regulation by the sphincter. [6] [7]

Stress Urinary Incontinence

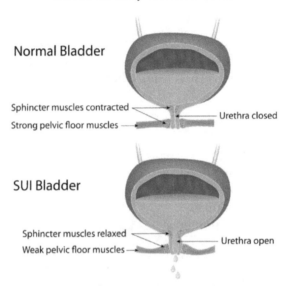

© Alila Medical Media - www.AlilaMedicalMedia.com

Figure 3 Above-Normal urinary sphincter endures high pressure enough to maintain closed with the help of strong pelvic floor muscles. Below-Muscles of the pelvic floor and the sphincter are relaxed, so the urine freely flows out.

Stress incontinence can be graded into three stages (Stamey):

Grade 1: loss of urine with sudden increases of abdominal pressure (coughing, sneezing, laughing, abdominal straining)

Grade 2: loss of urine with lesser degrees of stress, e.g., walking or standing up

Grade 3: loss of urine without any relation to physical activity or position, e.g., while lying in bed [8]

2.2.2 Urge incontinence

The person can feel a sudden urge to urinate, and if he/she doesn't react fast enough, the urine leaks into the underwear, which causes both hygienic and social issues. If the urination suddenly and spontaneously happens, this condition is called overactive bladder with or without urge incontinence. In this type of incontinence, a bladder doesn't function as it s supposed to. The detrusor muscle, which outlies the bladder from the inside, contracts more than it should, forcing the urine out through the urethra. The detrusor contracts improperly if the nerves that control its function are damaged due to various problems, such as diabetes mellitus, spinal cord damage, stroke, multiple sclerosis, discus hernia, or Parkinson's disease. This condition is called overactive bladder, since the bladder over-activates and over-contracts without proper nerve control. The bladder is emptied completely, letting large amounts of fluid leak out, without any warning at all. These urges occur even at night. Usually, the urge rises when hearing or seeing water running. This condition greatly affects the quality of life and is the main reason for admitting in the nursery home. It is important to take care of these people, since the urgency itself can make them rush to the bathroom, which can induce falling and injuries. They also have a higher chance of repeated infections and irritations due to wet skin. [7] [9]

2.2.3 Overflow incontinence

Sometimes the urinary tract has an obstruction and the urine can't exit properly. When the urine accumulates, the bladder enlarges, even if the person doesn't feel the need to empty it. This is called urinal retention because the bladder is retaining urine, and it can be a favourable condition for bacterial growth, leading to urinal infections. When the bladder capacity reaches its limit, it sends out impulses from the distended detrusor to the brain and back to the sphincter, which then opens allowing the urine to leak out. Paradoxically, a person may think that everything is fine because the urine manages to go out. This problem is called *ischuria paradoxa* because urine can flow and be secreted from the system, but the obstruction stays where it was, with only a part of the urine being secreted; the problem still exists but is ignored until the blockage is complete, and the urine can no longer go out. This condition is urgent, followed by pain and pressure in the lower abdomen, and he/she should immediately go to the hospital. The blockage could be from an enlarged prostate, a calculus, a tumour, a trauma or operation complication, or use of some medications that are called anticholinergics or antihistamines. [7] [10]

2.2.4 Functional incontinence

Functional incontinence differs from other types of incontinence because there is no bladder or neural disorder. It is mostly caused by problems with walking to the bathroom or sitting on the toilet. The person has functional difficulties with emptying the bladder properly in the bathroom. This happens to older people, and also to people with severe arthritis, back pain, stroke, paralysis, fractures, Parkinson's disease and multiple sclerosis, or amputation of the legs (because of diabetes or obstruction in artery flow in legs). They don't manage to empty the bladder in time on the right place because of their condition, weakness and pain when moving from the bed, or because it takes them a long time to get to the bathroom. Also, people with progressive neuropsychological conditions such as Alzheimer's disease and dementia aren't cognitively able to register the right time to empty the bladder. Sometimes the etiology is mixed. These people require everyday assistance from medical staff or family members.[11]

2.2.5 Mixed incontinence

Mixed incontinence is a combination of stress and urge incontinence, and it is most commonly associated with elderly people. It shares the symptoms of both urge and stress incontinence. Other than the conditions that separately cause each of them, factors included in the pathogenesis are thyroid gland disease, some medications, and diabetes. [12]

2.2.6 Transient incontinence

There is also transient incontinence, which occurs only for a short period. This happens during infections that irritate the epithelium of the bladder, which then leads to pollakiuria, the frequent urination of small amounts of urine. Caffeine or alcohol consumption can also provoke frequent urination. Transient conditions such as immobility, mental impairment, or the states that increase intra-abdominal pressure can also be the causes. [13] Transient incontinence lasts less than six months. Elderly people may often suffer transient incontinence because of delirium, infection, atrophic vaginitis, medications, psychological conditions (depression, dementia or delirium), excess urine output in endocrine illnesses with high blood sugar or high blood calcium, immobility, or stool impaction. [14]

3. Male and female incontinence. Are there differences?

3.1 Male incontinence

In general, men don't suffer from as many diseases and conditions as women do. Men's urinal problems are more likely to develop because of other diseases: neural problems, obstructions, or birth defects of the urinary system. Incontinence occurs mostly in elderly men. Most commonly, it is urge incontinence. If a neural problem is present, a bladder muscle, the detrusor, can't function properly, and then it pressures the urine out of the bladder, which happens involuntarily.

There are known triggers for urgent urinal incontinence. For example, hearing or seeing water drip or run, or drinking a small amount of water, submersing fingers into water, or even being in the cold, can urge a person to go to the bathroom. Anxiety, medications, or other diseases and conditions can make the incontinence worse.

Urge incontinence is, as we said, caused by neural damage, which may occur because of diabetes (where somatic, sensory and autonomic nerves are damaged by various factors, including high blood sugar); multiple sclerosis in which a process, called demyelinisation, develops on neurons (each neuron has its outer layer called myelin, which is damaged in MS); Parkinson's disease (the low level of dopamine in substantia nigra in the brain which is crucial to nerve functioning); stroke (neural damage of different severity, that occurs when brain blood supply is compromised); and others. When the neural control is damaged and disabled, the nerve signals are set off at the wrong time, and the bladder becomes overactive; therefore this condition is also called overactive bladder.

Men can also have all other types of incontinences. Stress incontinence may happen when a man suffers major head trauma, after a prostate operation, or with aging. Functional incontinence occurs when a man isn't capable of taking care of his hygiene and urination because of invalidity and disability. The causes that are most common are Alzheimer's disease, invalidity that requires a wheelchair, arthritis that can limit movement because of the pain, or deformities. Overflow incontinence occurs when a bladder is full but the problem lies in the distal obstruction: enlargement of the prostate, tumour, urinary stones, or nerve damage. [13]

Incontinence in men with enlargement of the prostate (benign prostatic hyperplasia) can develop because of the obstruction of the urinary flow, but also if the urethral sphincter localised under the prostate is damaged in an operation. Even after the operation, not all men are free from symptoms. That can be explained by denervation, supersensitivity of the bladder muscle, changes in collagen, increased sensory reflexes, or changes in muscle cells of detrusor, but also by direct mechanical damage that is inevitable during surgery. Studies have also researched the influence of total prostatectomy and radiotherapy on incontinence development. [14]

3.2 Female incontinence

Incontinence in women has a little different development. Studies indicate that approximately 50% of women who suffer from incontinence are suffering from stress incontinence. The incidence of mixed is right behind stress incontinence and then comes urge incontinence.

Risk factors that are most important for women to develop incontinence are pregnancy, vaginal labour, post menopause, aging, and surgeries. Childbirth can cause changes in the anatomy and physiology of the pelvic floor, especially if forceps are used to facilitate the birth. The baby's weight can cause weakening of the muscles of pelvic floor during the pregnancy and labour. The child's head pressures the pelvic floor and compresses the bladder. During labour, there can be injuries or weakening of the surrounding tissue of urethra. [15] [16] [17] However, Caesarean section isn't a protective factor against the development of incontinence, for reasons unknown. [18] After an operation, for example, a hysterectomy, it is more likely for stress than urge incontinence to develop. [19] In the postmenopausal period of a woman's life it is also more likely for weakening of the support muscles to begin. [20] Other risk factors are previous urinary infections, diabetes mellitus, estrogen therapy, high body mass index, parity, neurological disorders, loss of cognitive function, pelvic tumours, and stool impaction. [21] [22] [23] Women often consider that incontinence is a normal part of aging or a normal consequence after childbirth, and they comfortably wear pads more often than men do and don't seek professional help.

Stress incontinence is more frequent in women because their muscular anatomy is slightly weaker than in men. Also, estrogen deficiency has been proved to be connected with the development of incontinence. In addition, a condition called intrinsic sphincter deficiency is more frequent in women than men; this means that the sphincter isn't good enough and it lets the urine leak uncontrollably.

Urinary Bladder and Urethra

Male

Female

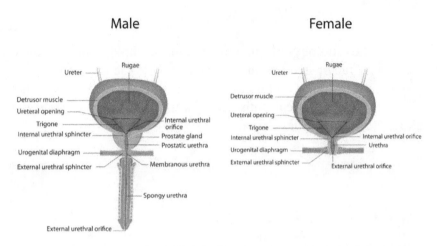

Figure 4 Structure of male and female bladder. Differences in size of bladder don't exist and it is approximately 500mL in volume. However, the urethra is longer in men than women. The figure shows the close contact of the bladder, urethra, and prostate in the male.

4. What causes incontinence and how does it develop?

The etiology of incontinence is complex but, in most cases, one factor is dominant. We can divide the causes into two groups: neurological and non-neurological. But first, we shall take a look at the historical pathway of various theories of how the stress incontinence develops.

4.1 Theories of development

4.1.1 Urethral position theory (Kelly, Bonney, Enhörning)

At first, scientists thought that stress incontinence is caused by anatomically weak structures. The factors that lead to weakening of the pelvic floor decrease the support of bladder, uterus, and anus. But then, besides the anatomical theories, functional theories developed as well. It was impossible to explain how the stress incontinence occurs not only with women who had vaginal delivery, but also in women who had Caesarean sections. That indicates that there is a functional defect; more precisely, sphincteric dysfunction. Early anatomic theories couldn't decide whether the weakness was in the urethra or the anterior vaginal wall. At the beginning of the 20th century, Kelly performed a series of endoscopic assessments and concluded that the bladder neck wasn't closing fast enough. The angle between the bladder and the urethra no longer existed because of the weakness of sphincter. [24] Bonney, in his public paper, concluded that the stress incontinence is caused by the downward movement of the bladder because of the weakening of the pubocervical muscles on the distal part of the anterior vaginal wall, which happens after the delivery. With the movement of bladder, it is more likely that urination problems will occur. So, he was opposing Kelly with his new anatomical theory. His opinion was that the lack of support behind the bladder resulted in dysfunction of the sphincter and stress incontinence. [25] In 1940, Barnes suggested that the cause may lie in high urinary straining forces or high pressure in the bladder, or in lower resistance of urethral sphincter, or both. [26] Enhörning used manometry (measuring of pressures) to determine which one was the reason for the leakage. He stated that vesical pressure stayed low against the high urethral pressure in a healthy urinary system. But, as the abdominal pressure rises, it equally affects the bladder and urethra. In stress incontinence, vesicourethral angle is flat, and they become as one, they both have low pressures against the high abdominal pressure, and there is no blocking of urine flow during strains and coughing or laughing, and the person suffers bladder problems. [27]

4.1.2 Intrinsic sphincter deficiency (McGuire)

These previous theories were widely accepted until new theories about the neurologic and sphincter dysfunctions were published. Some neuroscientists claimed that the real cause of stress incontinence lies in the neurological disorder, since the neurological impulse travels slower through the pudendal nerve than in healthy people. The pudendal nerve is responsible for control over striated muscles—the external urethral sphincter and pelvic floor muscle. The striated muscles are controlled voluntarily. The theory was that the nerves were damaged, causing internal sphincter deficiency (ISD), even though it has been shown that ISD can also be caused by muscle dysfunction. This theory concluded that there is not enough support around the urethra. The ISD is a condition in which the sphincter isn't producing enough resistance and isn't strong enough against the pressure in urethra and bladder. The causes of ISD are either congenital or acquired (surgery, vaginal delivery, or peripheral neuropathy). McGuire and later Green [28] [29] proposed the classification of stress urinary incontinence with degrees of weakening of the sphincter and its consequences on the system of bladder and urethra in regard to the pubic symphysis. This classification would be of use in assessing the bladder condition, symptoms, the specific type of incontinence, and the type of surgery that would effectively treat the condition.

4.1.3 Hammock theory–lax pubococcygeus back plate (DeLancey)

DeLancey hypothesized in 1996 that the weakening of pubocervical fascia can affect the spreading of the pressure on the bladder and urethra. The pubocervical fascia lies under the bladder neck and supports it like a hammock. If it is weak, the bladder moves downward, causing stress incontinence. This is actually a combination of the two theories of Bonny and Enhörning. But the pubocervical fascia isn't the only support to the bladder neck, so another structure needs to be damaged or weakened in order to allow the spontaneous leakage. Therefore, levator ani muscle weakness is also a factor here. [30]

4.1.4 Integral theory–weak pubourethral ligaments and other theories

Petros and Ulmsein proposed a theory that some factors combined, such as the effects of age, hormones, and medicines and defects of female pelvic anatomy structures may influence the development of stress urinary incontinence. They can all affect the weakening of the vaginal wall or its components, ligaments and muscles. [31]

Lose had a published a study about which region of urethra and bladder is responsible for the development of stress incontinence and came to the conclusion that there's a decrease in strength in the bladder neck and the mid-part of the urethra in women with stress urinary incontinence. [32]

There were also theories that searched for the mechanism of how the motor neurons that control the bladder and urethra and surrounding structures function in order to induce contractions and relaxation. The main neurotransmitters, through which a signal is transferred from nerve to nerve, are serotonin and norepinephrine. The afferent nerve signals travel from the bladder wall and detrusor through the autonomic nervous system, which is an involuntary nerve control system of internal organs, through the spinal cord, to the pons and the cortex of brain, and the efferent signals travel back, to the Onuf's nucleus, which builds the pudendal nerve, and in that way controls the external sphincter when intra-abdominal pressure is increased, so that it won't allow urination when it isn't the time or place. [33] If the damage is in any part of this system, difficulties with urination may appear as a consequence.

According to previous theories, stress incontinence is caused by anatomical or functional defects and dysfunctions, or both. More than one factor is included but, in most people, they are combined with intrinsic sphincter deficiency. Further research is necessary to discover other aspects of development that would create new ideas for treatment as well. Below is a table of possible causes of urinary incontinence.

Neurological causes	Non-neurological causes
Brain lesions	Outflow obstruction
Spinal cord lesions	Aging
	Estrogen deficiency
Peripheral nerve damage	Pelvic floor disorder
	Idiopathic detrusor hyperactivity medications

Table 1 Neurological and non-neurological causes of incontinence.

4.2 Neurological causes
4.2.1. Brain lesions

Our central nervous system is made up of the brain and the spinal cord. The brain is divided into the cerebrum, which is the largest part of the brain; the cerebellum, which is the smallest part; and the brain stem. The brain stem, which is located in the back of the head, has three parts; one of them is called the pons, which means "the bridge." The pons micturation (urination) centre (PMC) is located in the pons. If stimulated, the PMC activates the detrusor muscles contractions, opens the sphincter, and lets the urine out. With contractions of the bladder wall, urine is forced out and has free pathway through the sphincter. The physiology of neuro-urinary connection works like this: A distended bladder wall sends signals to the brain through the spinal cord; the signal comes to the pons, where the micturation can begin, but in order to provide voluntary control over micturation, the signal is further sent to brain. The brain sends activating or inhibitory signals to the pons, depending on whether the micturation is allowed to happen at a certain time and place or not. If not, the brain sends inhibitory, blocking signals, which are then sent to the bladder to lower the pressure and decrease the need for emptying the bladder. If a lesion is above the pons in the pathway, voluntary control isn't possible and the result is involuntary incontinence. This happens in strokes, brain tumours, Parkinson's` disease, hydrocephalus, and cerebral palsy.

4.2.2. Spinal cord lesions

The spinal cord is located in the vertebral column and is protected by layers called meninges. The spinal cord goes all the way from the back of the head, giving the branches and building plexuses for arms, thorax and its organs, abdomen, legs, to the bottom of the back, where it ends in the conus medullaris, small hair-like branches. It is divided into segments that are labelled with letters and numbers. The lumbar, lower back part, is labelled L, and the lower part, the back part of the pelvis, called sacral, is marked with S. The part of the spinal cord that receives afferent signals from the bladder is a sacral segment. In a child's development, the brain centre for voluntary micturation isn't developed fully, so most of the processes only go from the bladder to the sacral nerves, which then transmit the efferent signal for the detrusor to contract and the sphincter to relax, allowing the urine to flow. That is why children need time to learn to control urine until the brain centre develops.

If injured, the spinal cord causes the dysfunction of voluntary micturation. This can be caused by trauma, tumours, or discus hernia. The levels between L2-L5, S1-S5, and the coccygeal nerves form a structure called the cauda equina, which is responsible for sensations in the saddle area, and has a role in voluntary urination and defecation. The most dangerous state is *cauda equine syndrome*, in which a person loses the ability to voluntarily micturate or defecate, the sex functions are damaged, there is a sensory dysfunction in the saddle area, along with lower back pain and numbness and weakness of the legs. It is an urgent medical condition that requires emergency surgical decompression. Other conditions include multiple sclerosis, myelomeningocele, and tumours.

4.2.3 Damage to the peripheral nerves

The peripheral nerves begin at the sacral roots of the spinal cord. They are divided into sensory, motor, and autonomic nerves. The sensory and motor branches come from plexuses built from spinal cord roots.

The pudendal nerve is a sensory and motor nerve and one of the most important nerves in the pelvis. It is responsible for sensations on the skin of genitalia and it controls muscles around them. It's most important role is control of the external sphincter. It gives signals to the external urethral sphincter in order to allow or postpone micturation. In Kegel exercises, the most important thing is to contract sphincter and muscles of the pelvic floor, which are also under the control of the pudendal nerve. If the pudendal nerve is damaged during labour or interventions, that can weaken the muscles and disable the control over the urine flow.

The autonomic nervous system (ANS) is responsible for involuntary control of our organs. It is responsible for proper work of the heart, lungs, intestines, and bladder. The ANS is divided into sympathetic nerves and parasympathetic nerves. In the urinary system, sympathetic nerves keep the detrusor uncontracted and the sphincter contracted, thereby blocking micturation, and also they inhibit the opposite functioning parasympathetic system, which is responsible for detrusor contraction and the relaxation of the sphincter. The diseases in which the autonomic nerves may be damaged are discus hernia, diabetes mellitus, AIDS, Guillain-Barre, and tabes dorsalis (neurosyphilis). [34]

4.3 Non-neurological causes
4.3.1. Outflow obstructions

When there is a blockage in urinary tubes and the urine can't successfully be excreted from the organism, and if that state lasts for a long time, the toxins accumulate in our body, causing various types of damage to the systems. The blockage is called an obstruction. Against the obstruction, a bladder needs to contract more in order to push out the urine. It then causes a bladder to be overactive. There are several theories why the detrusor muscle contracts when there is an obstruction. Some studies say that there is a localized reduction of blood flow, which then leads to partial denervation, and improper movement of the detrusor, while others say that the bladder cells change their length constant, which affects the transmission of the signals from muscular cells to nerves, leading to abnormal muscle contraction. A third theory suggests that there is enlargement of the detrusor muscle in mass and strength, the bladder can't be properly emptied, and that these are responsible for sending out too many signals to the sacral segment of spinal cord, resulting in a hyperstimulation of the muscle, thus causing the incontinence. [14]

4.3.2. Aging

Aging processes include atrophia, a decrease in size, a slowing of the metabolism, and a weakening of collagen in the connective tissue. The latter is fundamental in the process of incontinence. The bladder structure is changing, the detrusor muscle loses its elasticity and contractility, allowing the urine to retain in the bladder. The residual urine can even amount to 50-100mL. [35] However, with the aging process the incidence of neural dysfunctions, such as dementia, stroke, and other problems rises. To determine whether the cause is idiopathic or neural, people can be tested via brain imaging techniques. In most people with bladder overactivity, signs of lesions can be seen in the brain.

4.3.3. Estrogen deficiency

At the beginning of postmenopause, the level of estrogen in the blood decreases, affecting a lot of organs and inducing the first symptoms of postmenopause: so-called "hot flashes," vaginal dryness, irritability, insomnia, and changes in menstrual bleeding. Estrogen influence on the development of incontinence is discovered after applying estrogen in small doses to women with overactive bladder and improvement resulted. This connects postmenopause in elderly women with incontinence and other symptoms of lower urinary tract (LUTS). [14] The problem with estrogen therapy is increased risk for cerebrovascular diseases and it can also alter the collagen metabolism; those are the main reasons that estrogen is not considered yet in the therapy. [36] [37]

4.3.4. Pelvic floor weakening and lesions

The pelvic floor is the main lower support for the pelvic and abdominal organs. It must endure the pressure when striate muscles of the abdomen contract while sneezing, coughing, laughing, lifting heavy objects, or running. When the pelvic floor is weakened in women, there is a high possibility of developing a problem like stress incontinence. It is not actually caused by psychological stress, as the name suggests, but by the stress or pressure on the weakened pelvic floor muscles.

There are three possible mechanisms for damage to the pelvic floor:

- damage to muscles
- damage to connective tissue
- nerve injury
- vascular damage.

Damage to the muscles has been the subject of many studies. The largest pressure is on the pubococcygeus muscle, but the other three muscles are also under pressure (in order from the highest stretch ratio to the lowest: iliococcygeus, pubococcygeus, and puborectalis) [38] and in pregnancy and labour, these muscles endure a large pressure to allow a fetal head to go through the birth canal. In addition, the use of forceps to facilitate the birth can injure the levator ani muscle. It is important is to note that there are natural weaknesses in the pelvic floor, called hiatuses, and they are openings for the urethra, vagina, and anus. If the injury is serious enough, it can cause all sorts of consequences, such as incontinence and prolapse of the organs. This is a mechanical injury to the pelvic floor.

Damage to connective tissue is any injury to the collagen, one of the fibbers in the connective tissue that provides strength, thickness, and elasticity. The biochemical composition and hydration of collagen are affected by hormonal influence during the pregnancy. Collagen is being remodulated, differently organised, and changed in length. That can have an effect on the pelvic floor for a short or long period. The more forces the connective tissue endures, the farther it will stretch under a constant pressure. Collagen structure in pregnancy can also affect increased mobility in the neck of the bladder, which leads to stress incontinence. Other risk factors are torn or stretched ligaments (the cardinal or uterosacral ligament). The damage can also affect the tissue of the vagina, which, after stretching over its limit, can be even torn. It can be damaged in four ways: paravaginally, centrally, distally, and cervically.

Damage to the nerves is the most common injury to the pudendal nerve. Most pressure during labour is on the nerves of the anal sphincter, but there is also significant pressure on the urinary sphincter. The damage is usually called mild and temporary, and it includes demyelinisation of the pudendal nerve. The mechanism is direct pressure, traction, and low blood supply to the nerve.

Vascular damage is mostly mixed with neural damage. The mechanism is combined and most likely is due to low blood supply to the nerve. [14]

Women are at more risk than men of developing stress incontinence and mixed incontinence. One study included 15,000 women, including women who had given birth and those who hadn't, and the two groups were compared. Women who hadn't given birth to a child had incidence of incontinence of 10.1%, while women who gave birth by Caesarean section had an incidence of 15.9% and women who delivered vaginally showed incidence of incontinence of 21%. [39]

In some women, there is a possibility of inherited factors, such as weak, abnormal collagen. A history of incontinence in the family also indicates a risk of developing it.

Other factors contributing to incontinence during pregnancy are the size of the baby, complications during the delivery, age, body mass index, physical exercise, and smoking history. [14]

In addition to incontinence, women have a higher chance to develop cystocele, rectocele, and urethral prolapse, which are consequences of a weakening of the walls of the bladder, rectum, or urethra. When women come to the doctor for this, they usually state that they had a feeling of something ''falling out'' [40] Not only the delivery, but the pregnancy itself is a risk factor for incontinence. The baby's position or weight affects it greatly, because they constantly pressure the pelvic floor over the long term. If the woman in labour had an epidural or a spinal block, it could be the cause of nerve dysfunction and numbness and the person may have the problem of distinguishing when it is time to empty the bladder. [41]

4.3.5. Idiopathic detrusor overactivity

When other factors are excluded, and we don't know what is actually responsible for the development of this condition, we classify it as idiopathic detrusor hyperactivity—cause unknown. Even though it is idiopathic, there are some theories about how the process occurs. Studies are concentrated on the function of the urothelium, the internal layer in the bladder. The urothelium responds with receptors on its cells on mechanical and chemical stimuli and releases various substances (adenosine triphosphate, prostaglandins, nerve growth factor, acetylcholine, and nitrogen monoxide). The urothelium is in tight connection with suburothelial tissue and the afferent nerves of the smooth muscles. They function as one unit. The function of the muscle is decreased or increased depending on the transmitters and substances from urothelium. If there is a change in neural transmission and substances, the detrusor becomes hyperactive. In some studies, myogenic dysfunction and denervation of the detrusor are the main events. They can lead to increased excitability and increased signalling among the cells of the bladder. The signal spreads through the whole detrusor and makes the bladder wall contract. But other studies have confirmed that junctions between the cells are decreased, not increased. There is a need for further research. [14]

4.3.6 Medications

Some medications may join with other factors in the pathogenesis of incontinence. The medications may induce or worsen the incontinence, so these should be known when diagnosing incontinence. Here are various types of medications and their mechanism of action on the urinary tract and also the effect of alcohol and its bad influence on this condition:

Alpha-adrenergic antagonists are medications that are commonly used for conditions like Raynaud's syndrome, hypertension, and scleroderma, but also benign prostatic hyperplasia. These can, however, induce stress incontinence by decreasing sphincter tone.

Angiotensin-converting enzyme inhibitors are very commonly used medications for hypertension, and are especially indicated in people with diabetes mellitus. However, 25% of people complain of a cough that begins with the use of this medication. Coughing is inducing the increase in intra-abdominal pressure, and provoking the development of stress incontinence.

Calcium channel blockers form a group of vasodilating agents that are commonly used for arrhythmia, hypertension, and chest pain (angina pectoris). Vasodilation comes from relaxing the smooth muscles by blocking Ca channels in muscle cells, and the same thing happens with the bladder: These medicines relax the detrusor and induce urine retention and overflow incontinence.

Diuretics are medications that increase production of urine. For obvious reasons, this isn't good for people with this condition, since the urine flow is increased, when they already can't control emptying the bladder, which can lead to stress incontinence of large amounts of fluids, or small amounts frequently, or can induce serious retention in the bladder if there is a blockage in urine flow.

Cyclooxygenase-2 selective non-steroidal anti-inflammatory drugs are medications from the group of non-steroid anti-inflammatory drugs that have effect only on the COX2 enzyme, a crucial enzyme in producing substances that are activated in pain and inflammations and are used in joint illnesses to relieve pain.

They increase fluid retention, causing night urination and functional incontinence.

Opioids are medications used for relief from severe pain. Their various adverse effects include vomiting, respiratory problems, and addiction. In the urinary tract, they decrease the sensation of fullness of bladder and increase sphincter tone. That leads to urinary retention and overflow incontinence.

Skeletal muscle relaxants are used for treating pain in biliary and renal colics, hyperreflexia, and muscle spasms. They can induce relaxation of the bladder, inhibit bladder contractions, and cause retention and overflow incontinence.

Antidepressants, antiparkinsonian agents, and antipsychotics are used for the treatment of various psychological disorders, depression, Parkinson's disease, psychosis, and schizophrenia, but can also inhibit bladder contractions and cause urine retention and overflow incontinence.

Sedatives and hypnotics, similarly to the previous group, are used for treating psychological disorders, or preoperatively and for relaxation and reducing panic, anxiety, and appeasement. However, they can lead to impaired cognition and sedation and then to functional incontinence or overflow incontinence

Antihistamines, anticholinergics are used for therapy of the hyperactive bladder, but in other cases, because they decrease bladder contractions, they can cause retention and overflow incontinence.

Thiazolidinediones are medications used for treatment of type 2 diabetes mellitus, and are also called glitazones. They increase fluid retention, causing night urination and functional incontinence.

Alcohol – isn't a medication, but it should be known how it affects and worsens the condition. Alcohol is a sedative, and a central nervous system depressant, with effects previously described; induces micturation and works as a diuretic; causes urge, overflow, or functional incontinence, or the combination. [42] [43]

5. What are the symptoms of incontinence and bladder problems?

There is an abbreviation, LUTS, that refers to any symptom in the part of the urinary system below the kidneys. The abbreviation stands for "lower urinary tract symptoms." They include:

- urine leakage
- frequent urination
- painful urination
- sudden, strong urges to urinate
- problems starting a urine stream
- problems emptying the bladder completely
- recurrent urinary tract infections. [44]

Symptoms of urinary incontinence vary, depending on the type and the pathogenesis of incontinence. Some people notice that the urine leaks from time to time, but others develop frequent and serious wetting of the clothes every day. The frequency and occasion are the components that sooner or later lead the person to the doctor. In stress incontinence, which occurs more in women, there is a small amount of urine leaking in certain situations, such as when a woman sneezes, coughs, laughs, runs, or lifts heavy objects.

A sudden, urgent need to empty the bladder happens to people with urge incontinence. This happens also during the night. The conditions we should be aware of are infections, diabetes, and neurological conditions. In overflow incontinence, there is an urge to empty the bladder provided with overactivity of the detrusor but, because of the obstruction, the bladder doesn't empty completely and there is always at least a small amount of urine remaining. This creates constant tension in the lower abdomen, above the pubic bones, with discomfort and the sensation of a full bladder. If a person can't move properly, is disabled or in pain, or doesn't comprehend that the need for emptying the bladder should be fulfilled by going to the bathroom at an appropriate time, that person experiences functional incontinence. If symptoms are combined, it is likely that there are few mechanisms. This happens with mixed incontinence.

A woman with bladder problem often isn't able to admit, first to herself and then to her physician, that there is a problem. It may take years before she seeks professional help. But it is important to note that incontinence not only affects hygiene and social interactions, but can also be a sign of other serious conditions, and it can cause old or disabled people to rush to the bathroom and fall. So, knowing the causes and risks, and with the first signs of incontinence, everyone should be advised by a doctor about further actions. [45]

In people with incontinence, there are also psychological effects. A person may develop depression and a decline in the quality of life. The main problems are the social stigma that follows this condition of not being able to fulfil one of the basic functions, which is the secretion of the waste products. These are often followed by the question of smell, hygiene, unpredictability of the incontinence, and embarrassment. These lead a person to avoid public places and social encounters, along with the fear of other people finding out, which then leads to solitude and depression and often guilt and lowered self-esteem, as well as the feeling of despair and hopelessness. These feelings and lack of motivation can be a serious barrier to therapy. [46]

Most women have a decline in the quality of life and between 25% and 50% of them have sexual dysfunction. Relationship problems appear in 38% of men and 32% of women because of woman's incontinence, according to one study. [47] If a person has a habit of exercising and doing sports, there might be a change or a decrease in these activities as soon as the incontinence interferes. That affects fitness and social life. [48] In the work field, consequences are also evident. A person is under constant anxiety of unwanted and unpredictable leakage and smell, which could lead to lessening of productivity because of the loss of concentration, loss of the ability to perform physical tasks, and frequent going to the bathroom. Other activities, such as going on a holiday, sexual activities, and sleep may also be affected. [49]

People with overactive bladder have greater psychological consequences than people with stress incontinence because, with stress incontinence, a leakage is recognized when it happens, which is not the same with urge incontinence. [50]

6. How is incontinence diagnosed?

6.1 Conversation about the incontinence

Based on the opinions of many physicians, a talk with the patient reveals 95% of the diagnosis. It is important that the relationship between patient and physician is based on honesty and righteousness, without discrimination, but with respect and dignity on both sides. A clinician shouldn't approach a patient with an arrogant attitude, but rather with calmness, patience, and readiness to listen. A patient should cooperate in return, in order to stay healthy or find out about the solutions about treating the condition, after which he can decide along with the doctor which methodology is to be followed.

The physician should, first, exclude organ-specific disorders; then determine the level of the condition's impact on the person, its frequency and severity; then prepare the patient for a visit to a specialist in a specialized institution; and, finally, prepare the patient for additional testing before following the progress and effectiveness of therapy.

The first information taken from the patient is age, what does he/she do for a living, has she been pregnant and had children, and then, most important, what complaints does he/she have, for how long, has he/she had them before, and with what level of severity; then, what measures have been taken to contain the urine. A female patient's most common complaints are that, after she gave birth to a child, some leaking of urine started to happen. It is important for her to describe the pregnancy and the labour, whether there were complications or prolonged labour, the weight of the baby, etc. If the woman has just started pregnancy, a physician will instruct her to do some exercises to strengthen the muscles of the pelvic floor. If it s a male patient, he is most likely to complain about difficulties in urination and urgency to micturate, as well as a constant feeling of fullness of the bladder. A patient is also asked about inheritance, abnormalities on birth, previous medical health and diseases, traumas, operations, habits such as caffeine or alcohol drinking, and medications being taken. For women, gynaecological anamnesis is of great importance. Some physicians use questionnaires in order to find out which type of incontinence the patient has.

The physician should ask how frequent is the urination, what amounts of urine are leaking, and are there any included symptoms, such as itching, pain, tenderness or tingling, that can be a sign of an infection. Other important questions are what colour is urine, how much liquid does the patient drink, do they drink caffeine or alcohol, do they have diabetes, and do they have any symptoms that could lead the physician to believe there is maybe a neurological illness. In older people, it is a precaution to ask them about the incontinence, even if they don't complain themselves, because of the higher risk. After the conversation, a physician should be able to know how greatly the incontinence affects the patient's quality of life and what are the expectations from therapy. [14]

Questionnaire

As we said before, the physician may use questionnaires as a diagnostic tool. To get as much truthful and objective information as possible, doctors came up with the questionnaire for urinary incontinence diagnosis (QUID) to be completed by their patients. The patient fills in the form, scoring from 0, which stands for NONE OF THE TIME, to 6, which is ALL OF THE TIME, according to his condition, and how much do the statements refer to him or her. Responses from the 1st, 2nd, and 3rd rows are summed for the stress incontinence score and from the 4th, 5th and 6th rows for the urge incontinence score. Below is an example of a questionnaire QUID. [51]

Do you leak urine (even small drops), wet yourself, or wet your pads or undergarments...	None of the time	Rarely	Once in a while	Often	Most of the time	All of the time

1. when you cough or sneeze?						
2. when you bend down or lift something up?						
3. when you walk quickly, jog or exercise?						
4. while you are undressing in order to use the toilet?						
5. Do you get such a strong and uncomfortable need to urinate that you leak urine (even small drops) or wet yourself before reaching the toilet?						
6. Do you have to rush to the bathroom because you get a sudden, strong need to urinate?						

Table 2 The Questionnaire for Urinary Incontinence Diagnosis (QUID))

6.2 Clinical examination. How is it performed and what is expected from the patient?

The clinical exam should include a quick evaluation of all organ systems: cardiovascular, respiratory, abdomen, and lumbar succession, and an evaluation of the nerves, muscle functions, and mobility. Sometimes, with a young patient, a clinician must have multiple sclerosis on his mind, so the quick eye exam is needed. Examination of the abdomen can reveal scars after traumas and surgeries or the presence of striae; palpation of the lumbar region of the back can be significant in assessing the state of kidneys, and palpation of the lower abdomen can be significant when there is retention of urine, for example. A neural examination may reveal sensory dysfunctions, depending on the part of neural system that is affected. If the S2-S4 are affected, a person would have numbness in the saddle region. Changes in walking and difficulties when trying to move the leg outwards and the toe upwards can indicate an S3 lesion. Numbness and reduced sensation in genitalia indicate an L1-L2 lesion, and so on. Also, reflexes should be checked (sacral cutaneal rexlexes-bulbocavernosus and anal reflex). Elderly should also be assessed in cognitive function and mobility through various speaking, writing, and drawing tests. [14]

It is also needed for women to take off their clothes below the waist to be examined. This exam may be performed by the general physician, but more often by a gynaecologist. A woman is asked to cough to see if the urine leaks out. Also, a doctor may include a palpatory vaginal exam and look for any bulges in the walls of the vagina that would suggest weakening of the walls and prolapses.

Pelvic exam

A pelvic exam may be necessary in the evaluation of a woman's incontinence. The examination is performed with a patient lying on her back, with legs flexed in the hip and knee joints and sometimes with the feet in stirrups. This is the best position for a doctor to examine pelvis, or vulva, urethra, vagina and anus. It consists of several parts. In the external part, the doctor looks for any rashes, swelling or some tumefactions. Then the internal exam is performed using a speculum. Thus, the vaginal walls and the cervix are visualised. Additional examinations could include a pap test and a bimanual examination of ovaries and fallopian tubes, but they are not necessary in this case. It is important to determine the severity of leakage under abdominal pressure. [52] The patient is asked to cough or strain her abdominal muscles and the doctor monitors whether the urine leaks. During the exam, the doctor evaluates the strength of voluntary and involuntary contractions of the vaginal wall (which is important to evaluate in prolapses).

Men are also supposed to be examined with inspection and palpation. Sometimes there is a need for a digital rectal exam, since the prostate is located in front of the anus, and can be palpated through the anus. A physician can then determine whether there is an enlargement of the prostate that causes the overflow incontinence. If there is a suspected enlargement, a physician should also do prostate specific antigen (PSA), a prostatic tumour marker.

Digital rectal examination (DRE)

The prostate is located under the bladder and in front of the rectum and anus, and that is an important connection that doctors use to examine the prostate. For the examination of the prostate, the rectum is digitally examined. A digital rectal exam is performed in a position that must provide relaxation, but must also allow the doctor to properly and as quickly as possible examine and evaluate the anus and the prostate. This patient might be on his left side, lying on the bed, with knees bent towards the chest, or standing up and bending at the waist to the front. A doctor puts gloves on the dominant hand, then applies a lubricant, and carefully inserts it into the rectum. It is important to notice the enlargement, symmetry, and consistency of the prostate from the front wall of the rectum. A prostate may be painful, which suggests benign prostate enlargement. This may be the reason for excretion malfunction because the prostate compresses the urethra. Just to be sure, if something suspicious is found in the exam, it is wise to do an ultrasound of the prostate.

The specialized tests—provocative tests

There are three tests that can be included in the clinical exam of a woman when there is a suspicion of urinary incontinence. The three tests are the stress test, the Q-tip test, and the pad test.

The stress test

To determine whether a patient has stress incontinence, a physician might have to perform provocative tests to simulate the conditions under which the incontinence occurs. This is done by positioning the patient in the lithotomic position (a position in which the legs are flexed in the hip and knee joints and raised above the body, similar to the gynaecological position) or in the standing position. The patient is then asked to cough. If the urine immediately starts to leak, it is considered a positive sign of stress incontinence. A more complicated and less valuable test is when the bladder is filled with liquid step-by-step and the patient changes position from lying down to standing up. [14]

When a physician has to determine whether there is lowering of the bladder neck, and this is why the leakages occur, he will perform a Marshall-Bonney test, in which he will insert an instrument (or fingers) into the vagina and lift the front wall. A woman will then be asked to cough or strain her abdominal muscles. [53]

Q-tip test

The Q-tip test is performed to measure changes in the angle of urethra and horizontal, which is normally in the range of 30°. After applying a local aesthetic and povidone-iodine, a Q-tip (cotton swab) is placed through the urethra to the bladder, and then carefully pulled out of the bladder and positioned at the urethra-vesical junction. The cotton swab should be well lubricated with anaesthetic to avoid discomfort. The patient is asked to cough or perform to strain abdominal muscles. The outer end of the cotton swab is normally moving in the range of 30°. Moving more than 30° is characteristic for women who have stress incontinence. [54]

Pad test

A pad test is used to determine the amount of urine that leaks and is not specialized to classify the incontinence into one of the types. A woman uses pads and measures them before using and after using. The amounts of urine on the pads are then added to get the total amount. Usually, the bladder is filled with liquid, then she places the pad, and does some exercises that might cause leakage. After about 10-15 minutes of exercise, the pad's weight is measured to determine the severity of the incontinence. These tests can be performed during a short or long period (24 or 48 hours). There are tables that calibrate the weight of the pad to the severity of leakage. More than 1 gram is considered positive for a one-hour test and 4 grams is positive if the test lasts 24 hours, where a positive test affirms the diagnosis of stress incontinence.

Karyopyknotic index

This test is used to determine estrogen deficiency, because it may influence the development of stress incontinence. It is performed by collecting a sample from the vagina with vaginal cells, which are different when they are not under the influence of estrogen hormones. [14] [55]

6.3 Urine test

After the basic diagnostics are done and the physician has at least an idea of what might be causing incontinence, urinalysis is a must. In the urine sample, it is important to see what colour it is, whether it is turbid, or if blood is visible. Other characteristics are bacteria, erythrocytes (invisible to the naked eye), leukocytes, pH, glucose, proteins, specific gravity, ketones, bilirubin and urobilinogen, leukocyte esterase, and nitrites. These can be detected in a laboratory test or with a dipstick test, which is used just to determine whether there's a more likely reason for incontinence (infection, diabetes, etc).

A simple dipstick test can quickly determine approximately whether there is a significant amount of bacteria, glucose, or proteins in the urine. On the dipstick, there are reagents that, in contact with a specific substance, change colour and show how much of that substance there is in the substrate, which is indicated as +,++ or +++. Sometimes urinalysis is not enough and a blood test is required. [14]

6.4 Bladder diary

A person with incontinence may need to make a bladder diary in order for a physician to determine how often micturation happens, what the micturation habits are, does the patient micturate during the night and, if so, how often. It is important for him/her to monitor and note how often in 24 hours the leakages occur, and did it occur when they were running, coughing, or lifting heavy objects. This should be of help by showing the patient what activities are provoking incontinence the most. He/she should also write in what they drank (how much and what kind of drink), since drinking of more than 2 litres of water a day, and plenty of juices, alcohol, and coffee can also affect the incontinence. If he/she has feelings of urgency for micturation he/she should note that, too. This diary is written for one whole day or for three or seven days, depending on the opinion of the physician. The longer the period, more difficult it is for a person to truthfully and objectively complete the diary, so it is preferred for the diary to be kept for as short a period as possible, but with adequate amount of information. Below is a standard-looking bladder diary, with empty spaces for accurate notation of the activities. [56]

Your Daily Bladder Diary

This diary will help you and your health care team figure out the causes of your bladder control trouble. The "sample" line shows you how to use the diary.

Your name: _____

Date: _____

Time	Drinks		Trips to the Bathroom			Accidental Leaks		Did you feel a strong urge to go?	What were you doing at the time?
	What kind?	How much?	How many times?	How much urine? (circle one)		How much? (circle one)		Circle one	Soeeing, exercising, having sex, lifting, etc.
Sample	Coffee	2 cups	✓✓	sm med lg		sm med lg		Yes No	Running
6-7 a.m.				○ ○ ○		○ ○ ○		Yes No	
7-8 a.m.				○ ○ ○		○ ○ ○		Yes No	
8-9 a.m.				○ ○ ○		○ ○ ○		Yes No	
9-10 a.m.				○ ○ ○		○ ○ ○		Yes No	
10-11 a.m.				○ ○ ○		○ ○ ○		Yes No	
11-12 noon				○ ○ ○		○ ○ ○		Yes No	
12-1 p.m.				○ ○ ○		○ ○ ○		Yes No	
1-2 p.m.				○ ○ ○		○ ○ ○		Yes No	
2-3 p.m.				○ ○ ○		○ ○ ○		Yes No	
3-4 p.m.				○ ○ ○		○ ○ ○		Yes No	
4-5 p.m.				○ ○ ○		○ ○ ○		Yes No	
5-6 p.m.				○ ○ ○		○ ○ ○		Yes No	
6-7 p.m.				○ ○ ○		○ ○ ○		Yes No	

Use this sheet as a master for making copies that you can use as a bladder diary for as many days as you need.

Figure 5 Bladder diary

6.5 Residual urine testing

When urine stays in the bladder, it is called residual urine. Retention can be incomplete or complete. Incomplete is when the urine can still be excreted, but with incomplete retention, which is considered an urgent condition, there is no way urine can be secreted.

Residual urine can be measured through ultrasound or post-void residual measurement with a catheter.

The ultrasound post-void residual test is performed after the patient has made an attempt to empty the bladder completely. He/she is then asked to lie on the bed. The test is performed with ultrasound. With ultrasound, a physician searches whether there are traces of residual urine in the bladder. The residual urine is measured by the ultrasound computer program.

The other technique, *post-void residual volume measurement with a catheter*, includes the use of a catheter, through which the rest of the urine in bladder is extracted. After the patient has attempted to empty the bladder, he/she is asked to lie on the bed. After disinfection of the area, other sterilization actions, and local anaesthesia, the nurse carefully inserts a catheter into the urethra. If there is a residual urine (post-void residual-PVR), it immediately starts to run through the tube. The tube is connected to a bag on the other end. The residual urine in the bag is measured. [57] The accuracy of the portable ultrasound scanner is 85-94% in comparison to catheterisation. In the catheterisation, there is always some urine left in the bladder. even after most of it is cleared. [58] But ultrasound measurement isn't flawless, either, so a combination of the measurements can be helpful in some cases.

The conditions that lead to retaining urine are an obstruction or low bladder contractility. But, it can also be present in urinary infections. According to the AHCPR (Agency for Health Care Policy and Research) guidelines, residual urine below 50mL represents a healthy secreting function, and over 200mL is inadequate.

6.6 Urodynamic testing

To find the pathways of the urine through the urinary system, along with its flow and obstructions, urodynamic testing is performed. The other tests measure the static function without testing the urination and simulating the situations that occur in real life. These are the procedures that evaluate the function of the bladder, urethra, and sphincters by provoking real situations. They help the physician to determine what is the cause of lower urinary tract symptoms (LUTS). They usually use other radiologic procedures, such as RTG, ultrasound, and imaging techniques.

Urodynamic testing includes several procedures. They are uroflowmetry, cystometric test, leak point pressure measurement, pressure flow study, urethral pressure profilometry, electromyography, and video urodynamic tests.

6.6.1 Uroflowmetry

Uroflowmetry is a non-invasive diagnostic procedure that measures the speed at which urine flows and the amount that is voided. No special preparation of the patient is required for the test, except that the test has more validity if the patient comes to testing with a full bladder. A patient is behind a paravan, in private conditions, and is asked to void into a funnel-shaped device or a special container. Patient is asked to void strongly, but not uncomfortably. During normal urination, initial urine flow begins slowly, then speeds up, and then finally slows down again. It is important that the patient confirms that the test results will be representative. Good cooperation with the patient is a must. While the test is performed, participant must not pressure the urine flow, but rather void as naturally as possible, and he/she will be asked to confirm it. The flowmeter, which is a special piece of equipment, measures the quality of urine flow and is connected to a computer, where the diagram of flowmetry is constructed. The diagram presents maximum flow rate, continuity, and amount of urine voided. This is used to verify if there are obstructions that don't allow continuity in voiding and to check the strength of the bladder muscles.

If the urine flow **increases,** that might mean there is a weakness of the bladder wall; if it **decreases**, it's likely that there is an obstruction. In decreased uroflow, a diagram shows a decrease in maximal urine flow and prolonged time of urination. Males older than 40 years usually have a maximal uroflow that is higher than 25 mL/s, and females usually have a maximal uroflow of 5–10 mL/s more than males at a given bladder volume. Uroflow diagram can be in a shape of **flat line** in patients with surgical removal of the prostate (post-radical prostatectomy), where the urethra is a little narrowed and urine takes a long time to be completely excreted. **Intermittent flow** time is seen in patients with obstruction of the urethra because the urine flows with interruptions. **Saw-tooth flow** looks gives a zigzag look to a diagram, meaning that there is probably a dyssynergy between the function of the detrusor and sphincter, while they are contracting simultaneously. If the patient had an obstruction of the lower urinary tract that has been removed, the hyperactivity of the bladder wall is still present, therefore the uroflow shows a great peak in the uroflow and it is called the diagram of a **super-voider**. [44]

Normal results are listed below. The uroflow depends on age, sex, and obstructions. Men's flow rate lessens with age. In children aged 4 to 7, 10 mL/sec is considered normal for both boys and girls. With ages from 8 to 13, the average flow rate for boys is 12 mL/sec, and for girls is 15 mL/sec. In the adult years, flow rate is for males is approximately 21 mL/sec, and for females it is 18 mL/sec. With aging, male uroflow decreases, declining to 12 mL/sec, and in women it stays at 18 mL/sec between the ages of 46 and 65. After that, male flow rate continues to decline, to 9mL/sec, and for female stays 18mL/sec.

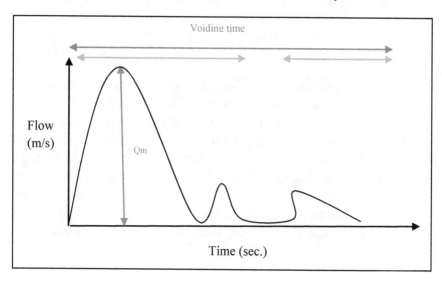

Diagram 1 Components of a normal uroflow

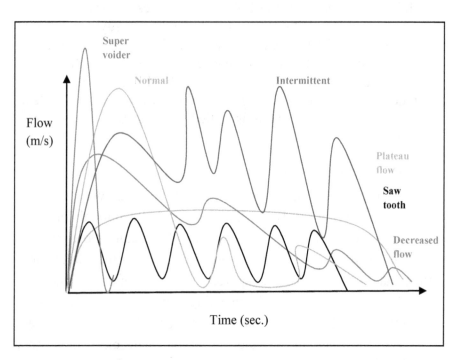

Diagram 2 Uroflow normal diagram and various other diagrams

6.6.2 Filling cystometry test

The cystometric or filling cystometry test is an invasive diagnostic procedure that measures a bladder's maximum capacity for filling. First, the whole content of the bladder is drained with a catheter, and then a special catheter with a manometer, which will measure the urethral pressure, is placed in the bladder, the rectum, or the vagina (to measure the abdominal pressure). The bladder is filled with warm saline solution, water, or radiographic contrast through a catheter. The patient is asked about sensations during the filling. Small dosages of local aesthetic are needed. The bladder is filled in approximately 10 minutes. A patient notes when the first sensation of bladder filling occurs, when the first desire to void appears, and there is a strong desire to void. The amount of liquid that filled the bladder is noted. If a patient has a decreased sensation, this is called reduced bladder sensation, and if the sensations don't appear at all, this is called absent bladder sensation. Sometimes a patient may be asked to cough or strain the abdominal muscles to provoke the detrusor muscle contraction. The results are defined by the patient's sensations while filling the bladder and detrusor activity. The detrusor may have normal contraction or overly active contraction.

First, as the bladder fills, the liquid takes up more and more volume of the bladder and stretches the walls. Pressure stays low because of the adaptive function of the detrusor, which allows it to stay low until the critical limit is reached. Any further filling of the bladder raises the pressure, which then proceeds to voluntary or involuntary detrusor contraction. [59] Detrusor pressure is the intravesical pressure minus the intra-abdominal pressure.

With cystometry, we can measure the amount of liquid that the patient senses, which is on average between 50-200mL of the bladder capacity, which shows the integrity of nerves, and correct function of the detrusor. The next sensation that the patient notes is the first urge to micturate, which is on average when the bladder is filled with between 200 and 400 mL. Also, we can determine the maximal capacity, which on average is up to 600mL. Differences between men and women don't exist; the myth about it came from woman's frequent visits to the bathroom, when actually, this has to do with habits, shorter urethra, and longer time to begin emptying the bladder. Low bladder capacity can be seen in some transient urinary problems, like infections, but is common in overactive bladder or a bladder that is damaged by neurological diseases or infiltrated. Increased bladder capacity is seen when there is an obstacle in uroflow, and in a neurogenic bladder. Here the bladder distends until it reaches its limits, and then the sphincter lets a small amount of urine out.

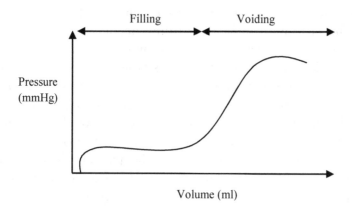

Diagram 3 Filling and voiding cystometry

6.6.3 Leak point pressure measurement

Abdominal leak point pressure is another method for determining the capacity of the bladder and the resistance of the sphincter to abdominal muscle pressure when straining (coughing or otherwise straining the abdominal muscles). A patient can stand, sit, or lie in a supine position. The bladder is filled through a catheter with radiographic contrast up to 100-150mL or even more and the patient is asked to do the strains or coughs. The pressures are measured. The leakage is induced by the strains and, when that happens, that pressure needs to be noted. An X-ray is taken at that moment to ensure that the leakage has begun. If the leakage doesn't happen, the bladder should be filled with more and more contrast until there is a leakage. The leak point pressure is the minimal pressure that causes leakage of urine. This method can also be called cystography, because it uses X-rays. If the patient doesn't leak at 250mL, the volume needs to be higher in order to leak but, as the volume is higher, the pressure is lower. Also, an obstruction in the urethra could cause the leak point pressure to be higher. This test also shows the state and strength of the urinary sphincter. A health care provider should repeat the test several times to check for consistencies. In normal sphincter function, it could endure a very high pressure, which is less likely to happen, and the incidence of intrinsic sphincter deficiency is high in the population.

6.6.4 Pressure flow study (voiding cystometry)

This procedure is similar to filling cystometry. To measure pressure during voiding, the uroflow rate must also be measured. This is usually done after the filling cystometry. The pressure is measured with a manometer positioned around a catheter that is in the urethra. The bladder of the patient is filled with liquid, and the patient is asked to hold the urine, until he/she gets the permission to void. With permission, the patient micturates, and pressures are measured (abdominal, detrusor, and vesical). Here the vesical pressure is the sum of detrusor and abdominal pressure and it rises as those two rise, or if one of them rises. If an obstruction is present, it affects the pressure (increased) and the flow (decreased). When it comes to measuring pressures, pressure is higher when compliance is lower, which most commonly indicates urge incontinence and overactive bladder. To affirm this, a health care provider can provoke urge incontinence by letting water flow loudly for the patient to see and hear.

6.6.5 Urethral pressure profilometry

This method measures the pressures in various parts of the urethra. Factors that influence the pressure are muscle strength and the abilities of other persisting structures to keep the urine from leaking. Even though the mechanism of the procedure seems as if it has a great diagnostic value, many studies have showed different conclusion. [60] The problem with this testing is that there are individual differences in the length and circumference of the urethra in people, and there are no standard values that can be used as correct referent values.

6.6.6 Electromyography (EMG)

If the physician suspects there are nerve or muscular problems that cause incontinence, the best approach is electromyography (EMG). This procedure uses electrodes placed on the surface of the skin or inside the urethra (local aesthetic is needed but, even though painful, it is not usually used in clinical practice). The skin is wiped with an alcohol pad and the surface electrodes or electrode needles are placed, depending on the location and the size of muscles. They induce an electrical signal and then transport it to the machine, which records the electrical activity.

Nerves coordinate muscle function and between them they build a motor unit. Muscles are excitatory tissue, which means that they emit electrical signals, which are here recorded by the special electromyographic sensor. If the nerves are somehow damaged, there is a disruption between the neuro-muscular connection, causing the voiding dysfunctions and the dyssynergy between sphincter and detrusor. The EMG test needs to detect the electrical activity of the muscles before voiding (in the phase of filling the bladder), while straining (high abdominal pressure), and during the voiding.

Electromyography can detect whether there is an injury to the pelvic floor after childbirth and it can also assess women with urinary incontinence. In these women, denervation and slower signal transmission will be detected on the EMG. Also, with women who had vaginal delivery, there have been reports supported by the EMG, that there is a significant decrease in amplitude of electric potential.

The weak points of EMG are that it is less representative where there is fat tissue and if the muscles that are tested are positioned too deep in the tissue.

The EMG results are displayed as near the baseline (which represents no activity or zero voltage), in relaxed muscle, and further from the baseline in contracted muscle, when muscle straining or coughing is applied or there is voluntary inhibition of voiding (suggesting increased muscle activity). The analysis of the EMG is done according to the phase in which the whole system is. When the bladder fills, the EMG shows increasing activity for a limited time in a healthy middle-aged man but an increase in activity in elderly men. During voiding, relaxation of sphincter muscles occurs and the amplitudes are low, except with elderly and people who can't retain urine, but the high amplitudes suggest that they are trying to retain it.

Women with stress urinary incontinence showed differences in the EMG from continent women. Continent women had higher amplitudes, and therefore better muscle control. [14] [61]

6.6.7 Video urodynamic tests

These are the most accurate diagnostic tools for evaluating a patient with incontinence. A type of incontinence can be distinguished with other methods, but a more sensitive and detailed diagnosis is best performed with a video urodynamic test. In these tests, X-ray or ultrasound can be used. If the X-ray is used, the patient's bladder is filled with X-ray-visible contrast; if ultrasound is used, then with warm water. The picture displays a real-time function of the bladder, sphincter, and urethra. This method can work under several channels: flowmetry, infused volume, voided volume, vesical, abdominal, and urethral pressure, EMG, and leak point pressure, so that it can allow many procedures to be done at once.

The patient is comfortably positioned on the ambulant bed and the catheter is inserted into the urethra. A rectal catheter is also inserted to measure abdominal pressure. The bladder fills with contrast that is chosen based on the radiological method. If X-rays are used, pregnant women shouldn't do this test. As with the other diagnostic methods, cooperation by the patient is essential. He/she is asked neither to withhold micturation nor to void. It is important that the sensations are reported. As the bladder fills, a patient may report a slight or strong need to empty the bladder and, if filling the bladder is painful, contrast is infused more slowly. If the patient doesn't have any sensation, that is also noted. Good cooperation by the patient is important because no methods can determine whether the voiding is voluntary. Also, when the patient strains, that can be noted only when the patient reports it. Patients who complain about incontinence when coughing or straining are asked to cough and strain. Straining gradually is better than coughing for determining even the slightest dysfunctions. After the need to void reaches a certain degree and limit, the patient is allowed to void, and the flowmetry parameters and others are measured.

Videourodynamics is considered a golden standard in diagnostics. It can provide not only the parameters previously stated but also the grading of stress incontinence and visualisation of anatomy. However, this method does have disadvantages. Dosages of radiation are small but invasive, and in pregnancy it is not allowed due to the chance of malforming the embryo. The procedure requires an experienced, well-practiced specialist.

In stress incontinence, the main task is to notice the state and mobility of bladder's neck, how and when it opens to allow the urine to leak out, and person's ability to stop the leaking.

6.6.8 Grading of the stress incontinence

Stress incontinence can be graded into three stages (Stamey):

Grade 1: loss of urine with sudden increases of abdominal pressure (coughing, sneezing, laughing, straining)

Grade 2: loss of urine with lesser degrees of stress; e.g., walking or standing up

Grade 3: loss of urine without any relation to physical activity or position, e.g., while lying in bed [8]

6.6.9 Other valuable diagnostic procedures

Cystoscopy - endoscopy (examination of the inside of the body by using a light, flexible instrument called an endoscope which is introduced into the body through a natural opening) of the lower urinary tract has aroused differing opinions on whether it is indicated for use in diagnosing urinary incontinence. There are, however, some indications of when cystoscopy is useful: to observe the function of the sphincter in normal and strained conditions; to assess the state of the bladder and its concomitant conditions; to exclude causes out of the urethra; during-surgery indications; to evaluate the sphincter's integrity after prostatectomy. Cystoscopy has no predictive value and isn't good in assessing the bladder function, but it is valuable when there are reports of blood in the urine of patients with urge incontinence, in which cystoscopic findings can give an explanation, or when there's a cause outside of the urethra, such as a vesicovaginal fistula, where cystoscopy can show the precise location of the opening of the fistula.

Pelvic ultrasound is a non-invasive, non-painful diagnostic procedure that can be an additional tool in diagnosing urinary incontinence. Ultrasound (US) uses sound waves that reflect from various surfaces to create a real-time image. The approach can be through either the abdomen or the vagina. Ultrasound is used, as we said, to detect residual urine, and also in video urodynamic tests. If there is a suspicion that there might be a tumefaction, kidney stone, or something on the wall of the bladder that interrupts its function, ultrasound can be of great value. The position of organs and the presence of leakage are also visible on US. Ultrasound is, however, of more use where there are weaknesses of the wall that create saccuses, such as cystoceles.

Cystography is usually conducted with video urodynamics and contrast. The bladder is filled only to 200-250mL I and is then visualised anteroposteriorly and laterally. This has proven useful in diagnosing stress incontinence. There are two types: filling and voiding cystography, but cystography can also be done while coughing or straining the abdominal muscles to provoke the movement of the vesico-urethral segment. That can be a sign of stress incontinence.

Intravenous pyelogram and urogram are invasive procedures that involve using X-ray-visible contrast infused intravenously through the arm. Several images are taken as the contrast passes through the bloodstream and secretes into the kidneys, ureters, bladder and lower urinary tract. This may be important in diagnosing the semi-obstructions and obstructions of the urinary system and residual urine. However, this cannot be performed on pregnant women.

7. What other conditions can look like incontinence? Differential diagnosis.

7.1 Differential diagnosis of various diseases with similar symptoms and/or signs

The diagnosis isn't certain if tests haven't been done that provide sensitivity and specificity. On the other hand, the development of some conditions is complex, so the symptoms are mixed and often mislead health care providers until the right diagnosis is set. These are:

Cystitis in Female is a very common disease in women. It is considered non-complicated and is treatable with antibiotics for 3-5 days. Symptoms are itching, pain, and discomfort in the lower abdomen with frequent micturation of small amounts of urine. The patient should be asked whether and how many times this has happened, and it is important in most cases to start the dosage of antibiotics, but at the same time to test the urine for bacteria and antibiogram. After the results of testing, therapy is continued or corrected.

Multiple Sclerosis is a chronic, progressive, immuno-mediated disease that causes dysfunctions in various parts of the organism. The symptoms evolve very insidiously and include sensory loss, muscle cramping, speech, walking problems, tremor, bladder, bowel, and sexual problems, optic nerve inflammation, double vision, fatigue, dizziness, and others. It mostly affects women between 30 and 40 years of age.

Prostatitis is an infection of the prostate. Prostatitis can be acute and chronic. Acute prostatitis is often caused by bacteria that may be transmitted sexually, but also through lymphatic vessels, the bloodstream, or surrounding organs. It manifests with generalized and localized symptoms: fever, pain in joints, muscles, dysuria (frequent, urgent micturation), night urination, hesitancy, weak stream, incomplete voiding, perineal pain, and abdominal pain.

This condition is treated with antibiotics. Chronic prostatitis doesn't cause generalized symptoms, but rather dysuria and recurrent urinary infections. Treatment is also with antibiotics but also analgesics, alpha-blocking agents, sitzbaths, hydrations, and soft food.

Spinal Cord Tumours can be developed from degenerated glia cells, neurons, meninges, osteo-fibrotic tissue, and other tissues in the spinal cord. In early stages, the tumours don't present symptoms and are detectable only by accident. Later, they can present with back pain, leg weakness, and bladder or bowel problems. Urinary incontinence, retention of urine, and leg paralysis are in many cases manifested late in the disease. To differentiate from non-neurologic types of incontinence, CT or MRI imaging is advised.

Spinal Cord Trauma and Related Diseases can give various symptoms and consequences depending on the severity and localization of the trauma, and whether there are motor, sensory, or autonomic nerve lesions (or a combination of the three). If there's a complete section trauma to the spinal cord, that will present as bowel and bladder problems (retention of the urine and constipation). Lesions of the lower lumbar and sacral segment also manifest as urinary and bowel problems. Cauda equina syndrome can originate from external or internal compression. It presents with retention of urine, constipation, flaccid paralysis of legs, and impaired sensation in the saddle area.

Spinal Epidural Abscess can damage urinary function by compressing the neurons of the spinal cord. This infectious disease spreads through the blood or directly from surrounding organs and tissues and with needles after invasive procedures.

Urinary Obstructions such as tumours or kidney stones can produce very intensive symptoms when they block the urine excretion. Lumbar pain is the most common symptom and it can progress slowly or fast, depending on when the obstruction closes the pathways. Also present are blood in the urine and/or repeated urinary infections and, as the obstruction progresses, symptoms and signs of renal failure.

Urinary Tract Infection in Males is considered rare in young males but, after the age of 50, these infections become more common, and are considered complicated because of the low immunity that comes with aging, and because they are usually the consequence of previous silent infections (prostatitis, epidydimitis, cystitis, glomerulonephritis, etc.). They can also become more frequent if benign prostatic hyperplasia is developing. With the obstruction developing, overflow incontinence also develops.

Uterine Prolapse in Emergency Medicine can present not only with a sense of heaviness in the perineum or something falling out from the vagina and pain and pressure in the pelvis or abdomen, but also with urinary problems such as incontinence, recurrent urinary infections, and difficulties with higher-frequency voiding.

Vaginitis is an inflammation of the vagina. It can have a different etiology in little girls and women. Women usually transmit the bacteria sexually, but other ways are also noted. The symptoms of vaginitis are a change in secretion from the vagina, redness, vaginal pain and irritation, and discomfort when voiding. [7]

7.2 Differences between the types of incontinence

Urge – A person may feel a sudden urge to empty the bladder. This is characterized by detrusor instability and irregular contractions and, if the cause is neurological, it is called detrusor hyperreflexia. In brain and spinal cord lesions, as in multiple sclerosis, there is a synergy between detrusor and sphincter that leads to urinal retention and renal damage. With the elderly, there's a detrusor hyperactivity with impaired bladder contractility (involuntary detrusor contractions), but they must strain themselves to empty their bladders (completely or incompletely). The consequence is elevated PVR (post-void residual volume), but also symptoms of obstruction, stress incontinence or overflow incontinence. This is often referred to as *overactive bladder.*

Stress – In stress incontinence, people complain about leakage of urine when coughing, laughing, lifting heavy objects, etc. There is absence of detrusor contraction or an overdistended bladder. The cause is urethral movement downward in women, or significant displacement of the bladder neck while straining oneself. The cause also may lie in intrinsic urethral sphincter deficiency (caused by congenital malformations of sphincter), and it presents more often in women with estrogen deficiency and manifests in older age or both factors combined are responsible. The sphincter can also be impaired by trauma, radiation therapy, surgeries, or sacral cord lesion. The sphincter isn't capable of holding the urine.

Mixed has the combined symptoms of urge and stress incontinence.

Overflow is associated with overdistension of the bladder, causing constant or frequent dripping of urine, but it can also manifest with symptoms of urge or stress incontinence. The detrusor is underactive or acontractile (caused by drugs, neurological conditions like diabetes mellitus, low spinal cord injury, radical pelvic surgery, or idiopathic) or there is an obstruction (caused by benign prostatic hyperplasia, or rarely prostate cancer or urethral stricture; and in women after anti-incontinental surgeries or in pelvic prolapse). There can also be neurological causes, for example, spinal cord lesions or multiple sclerosis where there is inappropriate and involuntary function of the external sphincter, which is supposed to act opposite from the detrusor (sphincter relaxes instead of contracting when the detrusor is relaxed).

Functional causes are outside the urinary tract and include dysfunction of the osteoarticular system, immobilization, or neuropsychological conditions such as dementia and Alzheimer's disease.

8. Treatment

8.1 Conservative management

Conservative management of the illness is an approach to reducing the symptoms and even healing with activities that don't use medicines or surgery but simple, inexpensive activities that were known to be of help for a long time, since the early beginning of the medical science. They include a healthy lifestyle, healthier eating habits, exercises, weight loss, and electrical stimulation. These methods are proven to be free from any side effects and a person can benefit either way.

8.1.1 Lifestyle

Weight loss

Increased weight puts pressure on the muscles of the pelvic floor, increasing the risk of incontinence and prolapses. The same happens with pregnancy. After labour, there is less risk. Obesity is reversible and, with the appropriate regime of exercise and diet, a person can lose a few pounds, which could help on the psychological level, too. Some studies showed that women on a diet had a decrease of incontinence. Forty percent of women who had lost 8% of their body weight stated that the frequency of incontinence episodes declined. It would be wise to review the eating habits, type of food, and the amounts of vitamins and water that a person takes in. Some unhealthy eating habits can induce constipation, which could lead to stool impaction and pressure on the bladder, which, again, is a factor in developing incontinence.

Bladder training

Some bad habits influence bladder emptying; for instance, when a person is accustomed to going to the bathroom before the bladder is full. This results in signals being sent with smaller amounts of fluid. Even if this is not the case, it is good to pay attention to when micturation happens, at what time intervals, and what amount of urine is voided. That is similar to doing the bladder diary, but with additional activities. The physician may instruct the person on training the bladder to make new, better habits in micturation and to postpone incontinence as long as possible. This training can be easily learned and can be done in the person's own time.

Incontinence can be mild, moderate, or severe. Mild incontinence is when episodes occur a couple of times a day, and with small amounts of urine. These people change 1 to 3 pads per day. First, it is important to measure the time interval between incontinence, and for that a bladder diary is helpful. Then a person should try to prolong it for 15 minutes. If the need doesn't come in that time, the person is advised to go anyway; that way the bladder creates new habits. Postponing voiding may be hard, but a strong will and motivation are crucial to prolong the interval little by little. Mild incontinence can be reduced this way. Also, Kegel pelvic floor exercises are allowed while holding the urine.

Fluid management

Intake of fluids is important for incontinent people. Some people think fluid means only water. But people also drink juices, sodas, coffee, alcohol, and energy drinks, which also produce urine. They also influence the habits of micturation (coffee is a diuretic and alcohol induces frequent micturation), so these should be reduced. It is recommended that the fluid intake should be decreased by 25%. But a frequent mistake is to significantly reduce the fluid intake. This leads to concentration of urine, which can be bad and lead to urinary infections, not to mention dehydration. The fluid intake can be measured by keeping a fluid-intake diary or using various Internet or Android applications that sum the number of glasses of water, juices, and other drinks per day. It is helpful to reduce carbonated drinks and caffeine and to eliminate alcohol.

Pelvic floor physical therapy

Many people have been advised to do exercises to strengthen the muscles of the pelvic floor. But most of them stopped doing any physical activity because it provokes the leaking of urine. However, specially designed exercises can be very helpful, not only in treatment but also in prevention. Strong muscle contraction can stop the leaking and elevate the levator ani muscle by inducing hypertrophia, the increased mass and strength of a muscle. Hypertrophia is a natural consequence of frequent contraction-relaxation exercises. The process of hypertrophia will begin after eight weeks of regular exercises. The exercises need to be done in a specific way, since they are used for specific muscles; resistance and repetition should be gradually increased. In order for exercises to take effect, motivation and persistence are crucial. Some lose their motivation if the progress isn't as much as expected or isn't happening at all after some time, or if it requires too much time, is considered pointless, improvement happens too slowly, etc.

These exercises are commonly called Kegel exercises after Arnold Kegel, who first developed them in the mid-20th century. They are effective if the incontinence isn't severe. They can be helpful to men as well as to women.

Kegel exercises. Kegel exercises should be done as instructed. The muscles that are trained are those that activate voluntarily when trying to stop the voiding or trying to compress the vagina or anus. These activate the levator ani muscle, which supports the pelvis floor. It is important that the abdominal, buttocks and leg muscles are not activated during the exercise. To prevent that, breathing should be relaxed and legs a little apart. It is important to do the exercises every day.

1. First exercise: doing quick contraction-relaxation exercises.
2. Second exercise: long-lasting contractions (10 seconds) and relaxation that lasts equally as long as the contraction.

Even when the exercises consist of long-lasting contractions, it is still important to take a pause that lasts as long as the contraction (here 10 seconds), because that is exactly how the hypertrophy begins. With repeated exercises come best effects. It is recommended to do 10 repetitions in the morning, 10 after lunch, and 10 in the evening. A person can do them wherever and whenever, as long as he/she is comfortable with the schedule. Doing exercises isn't visible to other people, which is an advantage. The exercises can also be useful in situations that need postponing of the incontinence (coughing, lifting heavy objects, etc.). The improvement is often noticed after a couple of months of regular training. It is good to check with the health care provider about whether the exercises are activating the correct muscles. Men, too, can benefit from doing Kegel exercises after prostatectomy. [62]

Biofeedback can be used to check if the Kegel exercises are done properly. This may be done by an experienced physical therapist or at home. Biofeedback devices are inserted into the vagina. They might have a monitor that works during the exercise and shows what muscles are contracted and with what strength. Biofeedback can also be in a shape of a weighted vaginal cone that comes in many sizes. In the beginning, lighter cones are used, then the weight increases; the period of contraction is at first shorter, then longer, and the exercise is done while standing. If a person succeeds in holding the cone in the vagina, the exercises are done properly, provided the cone is placed deep enough. It is best to read the instructions of the manufacturer or to talk to the health care provider. Some biofeedback devices can be placed on the abdomen to monitor the unwanted contractions of the abdominal muscles. If a woman has a cystocele or narrowing of the vagina, they shouldn't use these devices. Products for men are inserted anally.

8.1.2 Muscle conditioning without exercise- electrical stimulation

Sometimes the exercises are performed alone, for people with mild incontinence, or in combination with electrical stimulation. The aim of electrical stimulation is to strengthen muscles in stress incontinence and to induce relaxing in people with an overactive bladder. Electrostimulation may be performed at home or, better, at a physical specialists' office. The electrodes are inserted into the vagina or into the woman's or man's rectum. When the device starts working, the sensation is often described as being similar to doing Kegel exercises. When it comes to therapy for an overactive bladder that is connected with neural lesions, the electrodes are posted on the skin of the lower back, or on the lower leg (more about this later), where lies the tibial nerve that is part of sacral plexus, whose parts are the nerves for the levator ani muscle. There are, however, disadvantages to this method. Some women may experience severe pain and bleeding when using vaginal electrodes and the same thing is reported while using anal electrodes. When using on skin, pain can also occur, and there may be a predisposition for infections.

8.2 Medication treatment

Medications can be useful to some people. They are usually considered in therapy of an overactive bladder, but not with stress incontinence. Even so, a health care provider may recommend the use of anticholinergics, antimuscarinics, estrogens, and antidepressants (duloxetine). If the etiology is mixed, treatment is also mixed.

8.2.1 Alpha-adrenergic agonists

Alpha-adrenergic agonists are a class of drugs that affect the alpha-adrenergic receptors, which are divided into two groups, alpha 1 and alpha 2. These receptors are positioned on the surface of the cells of the heart, the central nervous system, the respiratory system, the urinary system, the skin, and other areas. They react to the presence of norepinephrine, epinephrine, and similar agents, which are called alpha-adrenergic agonists. When activated, they are responsible for narrowing of the blood vessels (in the brain, eye, and nasal mucosis) and contraction of the urethral sphincter, uterus, vas deferens, and bronchioles. Usually they are used for nasal congestion (stuffy nose), glaucoma, and hypotension.

These drugs can be useful in women with stress incontinence and in men after prostatectomy. Alpha-adrenergic receptors in the bladder neck, if activated, mediate in bladder neck tightening, which blocks leakage. This is helpful in reducing the symptoms, but some side effects could appear, including headache and vision problems, so they are not approved for longer use, and their use should be strictly controlled since they can be bought without a prescription. The most commonly used are pseudoephedrine chloride and midodrine.

8.2.2 Alpha-adrenergic antagonists

Alpha-adrenergic antagonists have the opposite effect of the alpha-adrenergic agonists. There are alpha1 and alpha2 blockers. However, the alpha blockers can be nonselective and selective (for alpha1 or alpha2). These agents bind with the same receptors as agonists, but they block the reactions and effects of activating the alpha receptors. Therefore the effects they are responsible for are relaxing of the smooth muscles, lowering the blood pressure, and improving blood flow.

They are helpful in men with overflow incontinence as a consequence of benign prostate hyperplasia. With relaxation of the sphincter, micturation is facilitated, relieving older men from symptoms. However, patients might experience dizziness and instability because of the lowering of the blood pressure. Therefore, they are administered in the evening when treatment begins. Most commonly used are prazosin, alfuzosin, doxazosin, tamsulosin, and terazosin.

8.2.3 Anticholinergics or antimuscarinics

Normal bladder contraction is controlled by the autonomic nervous system, primarily the parasympathetic. The contraction is mediated by muscarinic receptors of the cells of the detrusor muscle, which react to a neurotransmitter called acetylcholine. The main mechanism of action is by blocking muscarinic receptors and therefore inhibiting contractions in the detrusor. This is used for treatment of overactive bladder. Anticholinergics also have parasympatholytic effects on other systems as well, so the side effects are dry eyes, dry mouth, retention of urine, constipation, and problems with vision. The most commonly used are darifenacin, fesoterodine, solifenacin, tolterodine, and trospium because they have been proven to be the safest. During their movement through the organism, they are metabolized by enzymes P450 in the liver, which is important to mention because of the possible interactions with other medicines metabolized by the same enzyme.

The effect of this therapy has been the subject of many studies. They are the first line of medical treatment in people with hypercontractions of the bladder muscle. They are considered safe. However, they are contraindicated in people with narrow-angle glaucoma, myasthenia gravis, and ulcerous colitis. Other anticholinergics (not listed here) have been reported to affect the heart rate (by lowering it), and some may cause possibly dangerous torsade des pointes arrhythmia.

8.2.4 Desmopressin or antidiuretic hormone (DDAVP)

Desmopressin has a natural function in humans. It constricts the arterioles, but also has an antidiuretic function, i.e., the function of retaining water, depending on the state of hydration. Antidiuretic hormone is produced in the pituitary gland, in the centre of the brain, more precisely in the neurological area of the pituitary gland. It is then released into the bloodstream with short half life of 25 minutes. It affects the kidneys to retain the water and, as a consequence, urine is more concentrated.

People who have trouble with night visits to the bathroom and waking up at night to empty the bladder, can be helped with desmopressin, a synthetic analogue of human antidiuretic hormone, by disabling night voiding.

This medication is contraindicated in heart failure, hypertension, and conditions requiring a strictly controlled level of electrolytes. Side effects from taking DDAVP are headache, nausea, and hyponatremia, if drinking too much water. Because of this, it should be used only with the advice of a health care provider.

8.2.5 Tricyclic antidepressants

Tricyclic antidepressants (TCAs) get their name from their three cyclic rings of atoms. They were originally used as antipsychotics but, when their antidepressive effect was discovered, they rapidly began being used as antidepressants. They work as norepinephrine and serotonin reuptake inhibitors, which are unbalanced in depression. Blocking the reuptake allows these neurotransmitters to stay longer in the interneural gap and stimulate (excite) the distal cell. In depression, this means that they improve the mood, lessen sad thoughts, and increase motivation. These drugs can also be used to treat bladder conditions. Serotonin and norepinephrine affect the urethral sphincter through enhancement of pudendal nerve signalling, preventing it from opening at night. TCAs can also lessen the frequency of micturation in women with weakness of the pelvic floor. These drugs can be combined with anticholinergics. TCAs are contraindicated in pregnancy and breast feeding, glaucoma, enlarged prostate, diabetes, and liver disease. Side effects come from inhibiting muscarinic receptors: dry mouth, dry eyes, retention of urine, constipation, vision problems, and fever, but psychological side effects such as restlessness, hypersensitivity, and change in appetite can also appear. The problem with TCAs is that, after prolonged use, they must slowly be withdrawn. Withdrawal syndrome occurs after the intake of medication suddenly stops. The symptoms that develop are nausea, fever, malaise, headache, and insomnia. The most commonly used are Imipramine and Duloxetine.

8.2.6 Cholinergics

Cholinergics are analogues of substances that can enhance levels of acetylcholine on the synapses. They function in one of two ways: either as activators of nicotinic or muscarinic receptors, or as inhibitors of acetylcholinesterase, which degrades acetylcholine. It has the opposite effects of anticholinergics.

They strengthen the contractions of the detrusor muscle in women and men with overflow incontinence and a weak detrusor muscle. Cholinergics are contraindicated in gastrointestinal obstructions, bradycardia, increased function of the thyroid gland, epilepsy, low blood pressure, Parkinson's disease, and chronic obstructive pulmonary disease. Side effects are caused by activating the muscarinic receptors and include salivation, tears coming out of the eye, frequent urination, diarrhoea, vomiting and gastrointestinal pain. Bethanechol is the most commonly used drug, but it is not suitable for people with bronchial asthma, increased thyroid function, or Parkinson's disease, or for people who have had recent surgeries.

8.2.7 Estrogen

Estrogen is a sex hormone naturally produced in the ovaries. Estrogen can be useful in the treatment of stress incontinence. In many studies, it was suggested that the risk factor for incontinence is postmenopause. When the level of estrogen is progressively lowering, the pelvic floor muscles show progressive weakening, and these are connected, according to the findings of these studies. This is explained by estrogen influence on collagenous fibres, which lose their elasticity when estrogen is low.

The estrogen used for treatment of urinary incontinence is conjugated equine estrogen. It influences the alpha-adrenergic receptors and thereby increases the function of the urethral sphincter and the mucosal seal, and it can be of help with frequent micturation. However, many studies have concluded that the systemic use of estrogen actually worsens the incontinence and is responsible for developing new incontinence in otherwise continent women. But local application of estrogenous creams can be useful, if used for a limited period, 2-3 times a week. [62] [7]

8.3 Surgery treatment

Medical therapy has shown too many side effects, incomplete improvement, no improvement at all, or even worsening of the symptoms, so surgery has become a more common treatment. Lifestyle measures can be a part of a changed life, and people are usually willing to try it. It can also boost morale, because the person gives great effort to improve through exercises, healthy diets, and reducing smoking. The improvement is realistically expected only with those with mild symptomatology. But bladder training and Kegel exercises can be very useful, because of improved outcomes after surgery.

Surgical methods include various ideas of how to solve the problem of weakening of the pelvic floor, the major support for the pelvic and abdominal organs. A surgeon needs to be experienced, since the surgery is delicate, but it is a routine procedure for experienced surgeons. If the problem lies in a condition that can only be solved with an operation, such as a cystocele, there isn't any option that would treat the symptoms except an operation.

Operations for stress incontinence tend to solve the problem of the weak pelvic floor and opening of the sphincter. Some products are implanted under the skin to support the tissue, or a substance is infused to narrow the opening of the urethra.

8.3.1 Injection of bulking agents

Injection of bulking agents is a procedure in which a substance is injected to narrow the opening of the urethra, thus reducing the number of episodes of incontinence. These agents are actually the components of connective tissue. More and more used are bovine collagen, calcium hydroxyapatite, polyacrylamide hydrogel, carbon-coated zirconium, and polydimethylsiloxane elastomer.

The procedure takes 5-10 minutes and doesn't require an operating room. The patient is in the lithotomic position (lying on the table or bed with legs moved outward and flexed in the hip and knee joints) and gets local anaesthesia (2% lidocaine directly in the urethra) or a mild general anaesthesia or is sedated. Since this is an invasive procedure, urinary infection should be prevented with antibiotics. The bulking agents are injected with a needle, and the position of the top of the needle needs to be monitored with either ultrasound or cystoscopy. The substance can be injected transurethrally (i.e., in the urethra directly) or periurethrally (in the tissue surrounding the urethra). The transurethral approach is preferable. The agents are injected into the proximal part of the urethra, if periurethrally, in positions of 6, 10 and 2 o'clock. There is, however, some disagreement about whether to inject in the neck of the bladder or in the middle, and some studies support the middle puncture of the urethra. By injecting exact amounts of bulking agents, the lumen of the urethra is narrowed, which prevents the urine from leaking out during exertion. The amount of bulking agent needs to be neither too small nor too big and the procedure is best performed in stages. If too much bulking agent is injected, it causes complete retention and inability to empty the bladder. After the surgery, patients may have sensations of irritation, and some patients can't successfully micturate because of the urethral swelling for first few days, so a small lumen catheter should be introduced.

This procedure is especially helpful to women with stress incontinence who have intrinsic sphincter deficiency and for men who, after prostatectomy, develop the symptoms of stress incontinence. The bulking agents can stay in the urethra for a year. The risk factors are significantly less if the disinfection is done properly. The effective rate is only 40%, a lower success rate compared to other surgical techniques and this is usually due to the need for repetition because of relapses, resorption of the agent, or migration of the agent. New technology is researching the possibility of using stem cells as bulking agents, with the idea that the stem cells could initiate regeneration of the damaged or deficient sphincter muscle.

Women who have or have had urinary infections should consider other options, because this can predispose the stasis of urine and therefore increase the chance for introducing an infection or spreading an existing infection. Women who have any level of stress incontinence can undergo this procedure. If there is a sphincter deficiency, a patient should consider this operation, but it is much easier to do the operation if there is a simpler pathophysiology, such as a hypermobile bladder neck. If the deficiency is severe, it is better to implant a sling or bladder neck suspension as support. [63] This procedure is contraindicated in other types of incontinence, for obvious reasons: in urge and overflow incontinence it leads to urine retention. A month before the surgery, if the bovine collagen is used, a patient should do skin testing for allergies. [64]

8.3.2 Sling, male and female versions

Other approaches to treatment of urinary incontinence are based on the idea of supporting the neck of the urethra with parts of surrounding muscles and tissue. The first operation of this kind was performed in 1907 by using the smooth muscle of urethra and fixing it from a deceased person. Later, the fibres of rectus abdominis or fragments of fascias from the abdomen were used. The fascia that can be used are leg fascia lata and fascia of rectus abdominis, from the surface of the abdomen. However, this procedure can be done today with either the patient's own tissue or synthetic materials. Artificial material is used in TVT procedures (tension-free vaginal tape) and TOT (transobturator tape).

The procedure can be performed under local or general anaesthesia. Surgeons can use the patient's own tissue, allogenic grafts (from the deceased), or synthetic material. surgeon special should perform the procedure. The patient's tissue is formed from the fascia, the outer layer of the surrounding muscles, such as the fascia lata (a deep fascia of the thigh which is attached to pubic branch and inguinal ligament on the upper, internal side of leg); the fascia of rectus abdominis (the strong, straight muscle that is attached to the lower edge of the sternum and goes to the pubic symphysis, a muscle in front of the abdomen), and the anterior vaginal wall. The fragments of these structures are harvested by the surgeon and placed around the urethra. Cadaveric material from the rectus fascia and fascia lata can also be used, but there are negative opinions about this. Cadaveric material can degrade faster and can be a risk for bacterial infection, even though the procedure is shorter and brings a decrease in morbidity. Synthetic materials bring better results, since the operation is shorter, the durability is greater, and the incision is smaller, which lessens the chance for infections. Some show concern because the synthetic material implantation causes erosions and bleeding in the vagina, which is why there is a need for research of this complication and how can it be overcome.

The patient is positioned in lithotomic position for rectus fascia, vaginal wall, and TVT surgery approaches, or on his/her side with one leg flexed for fascia lata surgery. It is also important to be aware of possible infections, and all patients should take the urinoculture test and should be given intravenous antibiotics one hour before the surgery.

Surgery in women – Two types of surgeries are performed on women: TVT and TOT. TVT consists of placing a sling in a shape of U or hammock, in which the ends are not sutured, but just be surrounded by the connective tissue. There is a new procedure called mini-sling that allows even smaller incisions.

Surgery in men – In men, the incisions are made between the scrotum and rectum and the sling is introduced through the opening and attached to the pubic bone.

Surgeries performed in both men and women with incontinence involve placing an artificial urinary sphincter. This is actually a device that stays in the body and is manually controlled by the patient when he/she want to void.

In the *rectus fascia pubovaginal sling* approach, there are two incisions, one in the vagina and the other horizontally on the lower abdomen, above the bladder and the pubic bone. A patient is in the dorsal lithotomic position. After standard clothing and disinfecting procedures and catheterisation (Foley), the surgery may begin. Through the incision on the abdominal wall, the surgeon visualises the rectus abdominis muscle and harvests a fragment of the fascia. It is usually recommended to be 10cm x 2cm in size. The other incision is then made. The fragment, also called the sling, is placed around the urethra with the help of Metzenbaum or Mayo scissors and an index finger which is introduced into the vagina. The two ends should be on opposite sides of the urethra, left and right, and are pushed up towards the abdominal incision to be fixed to the abdominal fascia. There are rules to these surgeries. The sling cannot be too tightly fixed, but must provide good lifting and compression of the urethra. The incisions are then closed. For inspection of the result of the procedure, cystoscopy must be done to observe the state of the inside of the urethra. With the cystoscope, any injury to urethra on the inside can be easily visualised. The after-surgery complications may include injuries to the urethra and vagina and there is a risk of developing an abdominal hernia, because any incision is a weak spot in the wall, through which abdominal content can slip out. Some patients have problems with voiding after the surgery and they complain of the delayed voiding. In that case, it is advised that the patients do self-catheterisation for a limited period to help them extract the urine. Catheterisation will be more thoroughly described later.

Fascia lata pubovaginal sling is very much similar to the rectus fascia pubovaginal sling. Instead of the sling being cut from the rectus fascia, it is harvested from the fascia lata on the outer part of thigh. A patient is positioned on the side, with one leg slightly flexed. A surgeon harvests a fragment measuring 10x2cm. The incision is closed after a small tube for drainage is inserted. The patient is then repositioned in the dorsal lithotomic position and a Foley catheter is placed. Then the surgeon makes two incisions: one on the abdominal wall, in the lower part, horizontally, and the other vertically, on the anterior wall of the vagina. As in the previous procedure, the sling is positioned and the ends sewed to the rectus fascia. After the incisions have been closed, the surgeon needs to check the results with a cystoscope. Complications are the same as in previous procedure, but a patient is faced with another problem – leg pain that can be chronic.

Rectus fascia suburethral sling and *fascia lata suburethral sling* involve dissection of a fragment that is rectangular and smaller than in previous procedures, 3x4cm in dimensions. The patient is positioned depending on the fascia from which the fragment is harvested. The rectangular sling is introduced through the vagina and around the urethra like a sac and fixed on lower area of abdominal wall. After closing, a surgeon needs to observe the results with cystoscope. Complications are the same is in previous procedures.

A sling can be used a part of vagina wall as well. This procedure is called a *vaginal wall suburethral sling* procedure. After the patient has been given anaesthetic, she is put in the lithotomic position, the area is disinfected and a Foley catheter introduced. The sling is created from the vaginal wall by making two slantwise incisions in a shape of letter A. From here, the surgeon harvests a rectangular-shaped sling, 1.5x3.5cm in size. Then the surgeon makes a horizontal lower abdominal incision (before that, the suspension sutures were made from the connective tissue above the bladder to the vagina). The sling is fixed with the suspension sutures in four angles of a rectangle to that region. The surgeon then closes the incisions and introduces the tube into the incision for drainage. Then he inspects with a cystoscope. Complications are bleeding, bladder and urethral perforation, urethral obstruction, and delayed voiding, which requires self-catheterisation.

With synthetic materials, the surgery takes less time, and is less susceptible to infections and other complications. A *Gore-Tex patch* is used as a long or short patch, but the short patch has shown better results and less chance of infection. The procedure is more or less the same as previous procedures, except the sling is synthetic and no preparations from other regions are needed. The patch is introduced through the vagina and then fixed on the abdominal wall. Complications are urethral and bladder injuries, bleeding, and infections, but there may also be urethral narrowing, delayed voiding, and a need for self-catheterisation for a couple of months.

Tension-free vaginal tape – TVT is a procedure that requires special equipment: 2 stainless steel needles with polypropylene mash tape 1x40cm in size, a rigid catheter guide, and a TVT transducer.

The patient is given intravenous sedation and is positioned in dorsal lithotomic position. A Foley catheter is introduced. First, after local anaesthesia, the surgeon makes two small abdominal incisions in lower abdomen. As the surgeon makes vertical incisions in the vagina, local anaesthetic is injected in every layer before cutting into it. The rigid catheter guide is inserted into the urethra through a Foley catheter. By doing this, the urethra is fixated. After the mid-urethra is exposed, the surgeon makes a small incision on each side of the urethra. Through the left side, a needle is inserted all the way through the left endopelvic fascia to the abdominal wall incisions. The same is done on the other side. The catheter and rigid guide can then be pulled out. Before the removal of the protective plastic layer, the surgeon needs to check the results with cough test. The cough test is performed with a full bladder (250mL of saline). A cystoscopic exam needs to be performed during that testing. While the patient coughs, a surgeon pulls the ends of the tape upward to prevent leakage. If the position is correct, the plastic sheath can be removed, and the ends of the tape are cut bellow to the skin. Complications include urethral and bladder injury, infections, and abscess, but they are rare. A surgeon should observe the patient for urethral obstruction.

Transobturator tape (Monarch) sling (TOT) is similar to TVT, except that the incisions are made on the medial portion of the obturator canal rather than on the lower abdomen. The equipment needed for this procedure is a mesh polypropylene tape, stainless steel trocars spirally shaped with a plastic handle, and a steel-winged guide. The patient receives sedative intravenously, and positions in dorsal lithotomic position. A Foley catheter is introduced. The difference from TVT is the place where the trocar will exit. The anterior vaginal wall is cut after the injection of local anaesthetics, and the mid-urethra is visualised. Much as in TVT, the surgeon makes two incisions, on left and right side of urethra. Through them, the trocars are introduced. The obturator canal is where the trocar will exit. It is an opening in the pelvis bone between two branches of the pubic bone. Through those openings, the sling is introduced from each side. The surgeon can detect the location of that canal by palpating the tendon of the adductor longus muscle and lower pubic branch, at the point where the pelvis meets the leg. Below the crossing of the two, he/she should make a small incision. The steel-winged guide can ease the insertion through incisions left and right of the urethra. When the tip of trocar reaches the obturator incisions, the tape is attached and the spiral trocar is inverted back inside along with the mesh tape. This is done on the other side, as well. The surgeon should perform the cough test and cystoscopy to check the results and properly position the tape.

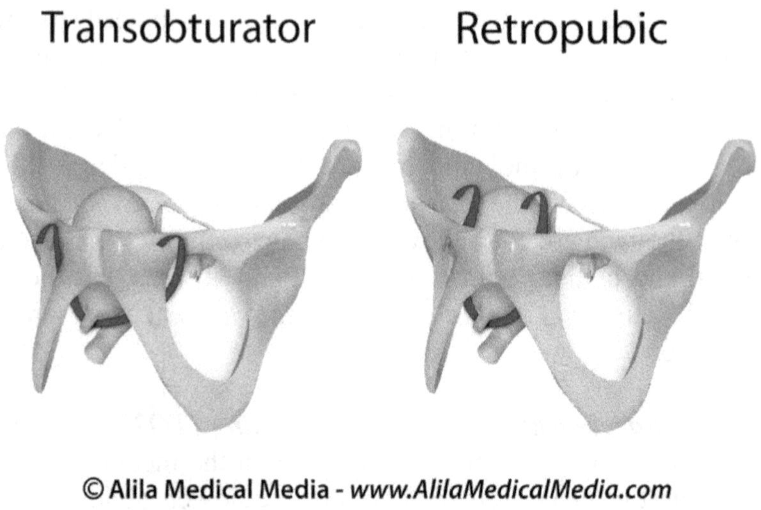

Transobturator   Retropubic

© Alila Medical Media - www.AlilaMedicalMedia.com

Figure 6 TOT and TVT procedures

Mini-sling is a single vaginal incision procedure that uses a slim needle that is inserted to the left and right of the urethra without cutting through the skin of the groin or abdomen. The purpose of single-cut procedures is to minimize complications. The types of mini-sling are TVT secure, U configuration, and mini-arc. Further research is needed to determine whether the outcome is better and the rate of complications is less.

For men with stress incontinence, the golden standard is to perform the artificial urinary sphincter placement but, when that is not possible, other options for men are *InVance* and *AdVance*. If a man has a mild degree of stress incontinence due to sphincter dysfunction after prostatectomy, these procedures are recommended, and indications for AMS800 (artificial urinary sphincter) are only for men with severe sphincter problems. These procedures are simple, take a half-hour to perform, and include sling insertion through an incision made between rectum and scrotum. The surgeon opens the tissue until he/she sees the bulbocavernosus muscle. It is usually done with spinal anaesthesia. For AdVance, the surgeon makes two incisions in the obturator foramen and through them inserts the spiral needle; when the needle perforates to the bulbocavernosus muscle, the surgeon connects the sling tape to it, and the needle is pulled back out with the tape. The same is done on the other side. The sling is sutured to the bulb of the urethra. But it is first pulled upward and tightened, without creating an obstruction. This is when cystoscopy should be done to check the result. After the sling is in the proper place, the incisions are closed. InVance surgery includes fixation to the pubic bones, while positioning the sling on the frontal side of urethra.

These procedures have become more and more popular, but because of the delicacy of the procedure and the dense network of blood vessels and nerves, a surgeon must choose the type of the procedure in which he/she is more experienced in. Sling procedures are minimally invasive and therefore the operation takes little time and is rarely followed by complications. All degrees of stress incontinence can be treated with sling operations. This operation can be performed in women with stress urinary incontinence and men after prostatectomy if they can't control their urinary sphincter. The procedures are different, but the idea is the same. Slings are contraindicated in patients with urge and mixed, predominantly urge, incontinence. If the detrusor muscle shows weaknesses, the operation is also not recommended because of the risk of the retention. [65] [66]

8.3.3 Bladder neck suspension, Burch procedure, open or laparoscopic

Stress incontinence can be caused either by the displacement of the ureterovesical junction extra-abdominally or by intrinsic sphincter deficiency. This procedure showed good results in changing the position of the ureterovesical junction by suspending the bladder neck. The procedure is called the Burch procedure or retropubic urethropexy. Another, similar procedure is called Marshall-Marchetti-Krantz (MMK), but the Burch procedure is performed more often. It can be done as open or laparoscopic surgery. Since open surgery brings greater risk for infections, a longer stay in the hospital and monitoring, and higher morbidity in general, laparoscopic surgery is recommended in most situations. However, laparoscopy requires good knowledge, practice, and experience on the part of the surgeon because, if those are not present, laparoscopy can create even greater morbidity than open surgery.

This procedure doesn't involve implanting the patient's own tissue or foreign, synthetic material as grafts in the body. That's why some patients prefer this operation. In comparison, sling operations have bigger success in treating stress incontinence, but also have higher morbidity (erosions, voiding problems, etc.) of 63% compared to 49% in the Burch procedure. In the sling procedure, the chance of developing voiding dysfunction is 14%, against 2% in Burch surgery. (67) When comparing laparoscopic and open surgery approach, laparoscopic procedure showed a surprisingly lower success rate then open, but higher longevity after 5 years from surgery.

The aim of these procedures is to reposition the ureterovesical junction and the upper part of the urethra in the abdomen. The procedure is done when sling surgery is complicated (erosions), when the vaginal approach can't be performed, when a patient doesn't want any graft implantation, and when conservative measures don't improve the condition. It's contraindicated to conduct this procedure in severe urinary stress incontinence, when a patient has a cystocele or rectocele, in women who plan pregnancy, and in patients who are not allowed, because of their general condition, to be under general anaesthesia or to undergo open procedure or laparoscopy.

A patient is in the supine position, with legs rotated outwards to allow the vaginal approach. The procedure is performed with general anaesthesia, and rarely with spinal anaesthesia. A Foley catheter is placed. In the open surgery, the incision can be either lower midline abdominal-vertical or Pfannenstiel-horizontal in the lower abdomen. The rectus fascia is cut and the rectus muscles pulled outwards. The surgeon must carefully approach the area around the bladder and avoid cutting the peritoneum. The bladder can be filled with saline solution, to facilitate the recognizing of the bladder neck. The bladder is pulled to the back and the fascias around the bladder are sewed to Cooper's ligament, which lies on the superior branch of the pubic bone. It is recommended that 2-4 sutures be made on each side. Here also it may be helpful to perform cystoscopy to check the urethra and bladder for injuries. It is good to place a tube coming from the space behind the bladder (the space of Retzius) to drain the eventual blood. The patient must stay in the hospital for two days and recovery takes a couple of weeks.

Laparoscopic surgery can be performed intra-abdominally or extra-peritoneally. The procedure is similar, except the surgeon uses smaller incisions to approach the organs and fascia. Complications of surgery are from general anaesthesia; as for local complications, infections, hernia, bleeding, difficulty in voiding, retention of urine, or new onset incontinence can occur. A more specific complication to this surgery is groin or leg pain as part of the post-colposuspension syndrome. [68]

8.3.4 Artificial urinary sphincter

In males with stress incontinence who have undergone prostatectomy surgery, there are not many options for treating the new incontinence. Medications bring no improvement. The standard surgical procedure involves an *artificial urinary sphincter (AUS)*. The AMS 800 device is the artificial urinary sphincter that is most commonly used. The parts of the AMS 800 are: pressure-regulating balloon, inflatable cuff, and a control pump. The balloon has two functions: to regulate pressure and to be a reservoir for fluid. It is usually placed in the lower abdomen, the cuff is placed around the urethra, and the control pump is in subcutaneous tissue of scrotum (or labia, in the outer genitalia of a female patient, since this operation can also be done in women). The control pump consists of one-directional valves, a delayed-fill resistor, a locking mechanism, and a deflate pump. To void, a patient must unlock the pump and the sphincter by palpating the device in scrotum. That triggers the opening of the cuff. The urine flows until the bladder is empty. The cuff is then automatically inflated, closing the urethra again. This mechanism is proven to give good results but, even so, some patients are not satisfied, or the incontinence again occurs and that is usually connected to improper use or dysfunction of the pump or silicone tubes that deteriorate with time. [69]

8.4 Other procedures

8.4.1 Sacral neuromodulation

This procedure is indicated in severe overactive bladder, overflow incontinence, urinary retention, frequent urination, or any other kind of neurological disorder that compromises urination. Implanting a pacemaker-like device close to the sacrum and nerves showed good results in patients with neurological dysfunctions of the bladder. It brought improvement in patients with urge incontinence and can be implanted in women and men. if there has been no improvement with conservative methods of treatment, sacral neuromodulation is recommended. What is good with operations like this is that a patient can go through a test phase by connecting the wire to the external device, then observing and analyzing whether it is a good option for treatment or not. The device sends electrical impulses to an area near the sacral nerves to modulate the start of the action potential, thus modulating the function of the levator ani, sphincters, bladder capacity, etc.

A test phase is conducted under general or local anaesthesia, with the patient being awake and able to confirm the sensations. The patient is in prone position, with lower back exposed, and the surgeon makes an incision just above the sacrum, on the lower back. After localising the middle part of the sacrum, the surgeon introduces a needle in S3 openings on both sides. To check for accurate positioning, a surgeon needs to stimulate the nerves near the needles. This induces contractions of the levator ani muscle and also flexing of the foot. Any other action shows that the needle is not in the appropriate position. Now, wires can be inserted through the needles. A wire is connected to the external device, the pacemaker, and a person spends five to seven days testing the effect of neuromodulation. If there is improvement, the patient is scheduled for surgery to implant the pacemaker inside the body. This time, a patient is under general anaesthesia, again in the prone position. A pacemaker-like device is implanted in the deep subcutaneous tissue in the buttocks. Before and after the procedure a patient needs to be well informed and educated about the use of the device, and how he/she can manually adjust the voiding, frequency, etc. The device's battery needs to be changed every three years. Risk factors with this procedure include infections, moving of the device, pain. It is contraindicated for the device to be implanted in a patient who has obstructive diseases of the urinary tract as benign prostatic hyperplasia, prostatic cancer, or urethral stricture. Also, if the test phase proved to be ineffective, the device can't be permanently implanted. A patient who can't understand how to use the device and what is it for, and whose cognitive abilities are not adequate for using the device, also shouldn't have this operation. After all, a patient needs to know what activities and procedures to avoid when having an implanted neuromodulator. He/she can't undergo diathermy treatment (a type of physical therapy with heating), or go scuba diving and do stretching, bending, or twisting exercises, because they can damage the device. The device interferes with a cardiac pacemaker and can cause injuries if the patient undergoes some diagnostic procedures, such as an MRI. [70]

Even though a patient needs a subtle change in activities and there are some adverse effects, a Cochrane study proved that the improvement is significantly greater than with no procedure at all. [14] But, even so, the device and its frequent malfunctioning must be under constant attention, not to mention how it affects the quality of life.

8.4.2 Percutaneous tibial nerve stimulation

Previously we said that, if the S3 nerve action is modulated, the levator ani muscle contracts but that also causes the plantar flexion. The tibial nerve goes through the leg and it consists of nerves from L4 to S3. These roots from the spine bring sensory nerves to the bladder and pelvic floor, and also to the leg. That tells us that the same nerve is responsible for both actions. This characteristic is used to improve the condition from another approach.

In this procedure, a wire (electrode and needle) is inserted into the tibial nerve, which is located on the inner side of the lower leg, a little above the ankle joint. The wire is connected to an external device that sends the electrical pulses; this device is positioned on the surface of the arch of the foot. The stimulation of 0.5-0.9mA and 20Hz goes through the tibial nerve to the sacral nerve, where it modulates the signals that go to the bladder and with that controls its function and can affect the incontinence in an overactive bladder. The treatment usually takes 30 minutes and is conducted once a week for 12 weeks. The research shows that the tibial neuromodulation is less invasive than sacral neuromodulation. Side effects include pain, migration, infection, dysfunctions with the device, and sensations of mild electrical shock. These devices need a battery change every five years.

Since the main treatment of this patient is medical, with anticholinergics, this device is indicated when there is no submission to these drugs. [71] The comfortable aspect of this device is that a patient can sit and relax during the treatment. The effectiveness is between 60% and 80% and the patients who develop improvement can maintain that improved condition by coming to the health care provider's office for occasional treatments. [72]

8.4.3 Injection of botulinum toxin

Over the years, scientists developed various uses for botulinum toxin. Botulinum toxin A (Botox) is approved for use for overactive bladder. Overactive bladder is a condition of inadequate contractions of the bladder because of neurological lesions. To slow and modulate the contraction, a form of neurotoxin can be useful because it blocks neuromuscular transmission and inhibits the function of acetylcholine. The whole procedure can be done under local or general anaesthesia with the help of a rigid or flexible cystoscope. As with any other procedure, a surgeon must be assured of no infections before and after the procedure. Therefore, systemic antibiotics are administered before it is begun. Botulinum toxin A is injected through the endoscope. But bladder is first filled with a saline solution for better visualisation. The toxin is injected in 30 places under the epithelial tissue of bladder, into the muscle. It is important, however, not to inject it in the area of bladder trigonum. Sometimes methylene blue or indigo carmine is added to the toxin solution to mark the previously injected places. A surgeon starts in the midline to the left and then goes to the right. The total effect occurs after seven days so, if the patient used any therapy, he/she shouldn't discontinue it yet.

Complications and side effects include generalized weakness, problems with swallowing, double and blurred vision (generalized effects of botulinum toxin), but no serious side effects like respiratory paralysis were reported. More often, patients complained of pain in the places of injection, blood in the urine, increased residual urine, and infections. Sometimes, it is recommended to do the self-catheterisation because of the urine retention. Patients who suffer from myasthenia gravis are not advised to undergo this procedure, since it can worsen their condition. There is a very small chance to develop an overdose from Botox injection, but the doses used are 10-100 times less than a lethal dose. Higher dosages are proven to be more effective for treatment of incontinence but with more side effects. It is not considered the first line of treatment, but its effects are supported by various studies. One large study showed improvement with 73% of patients who were administered with Botox. When a patient shows no improvement with conservative treatment, this procedure can be more helpful. [73] [74] [75]

9. Incontinence products

Before the treatment is determined or surgery is performed, patients have to wait for a certain time to deal with the problem of incontinence in their everyday lives by themselves. Sometimes the products are combined with treatment. If a therapy isn't successful or is partially successful, a person might have to use the products to lessen the symptoms. Incontinence products are carefully designed to provide maximum hygiene and comfort and to improve the quality of life. They usually collect urine and neutralize its contents and they should be comfortable to wear, invisible to other people, and easy to use. These products vary, depending on the group that the product is designed for. Products are different for men, women, and people of different ages; other factors are the type and severity of leakage. There are three types of products: for retention (to empty the bladder), for incontinence (to collect urine), and for toileting (aids for easier toilet use). A health care provider needs to determine which product the person needs in order to completely cover his/hers condition. Factors considered are gender, age, type and frequency of incontinence, cognitive abilities, mobility, work status, personal priorities, and different occasions.

The classification of products:

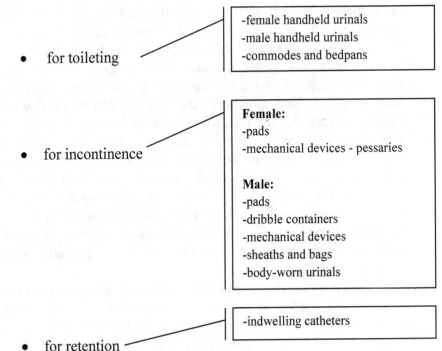

- for toileting
  - -female handheld urinals
  - -male handheld urinals
  - -commodes and bedpans

- for incontinence
  - **Female:**
  - -pads
  - -mechanical devices - pessaries

  - **Male:**
  - -pads
  - -dribble containers
  - -mechanical devices
  - -sheaths and bags
  - -body-worn urinals

- for retention
  - -indwelling catheters

9.1 Products for absorption pads and other products

Products for absorption, called pads, are used every day, worn on the body. Underpads are absorptive products that are placed under the person. Either way, they come in all shapes and sizes to provide a maximum area of absorption, according to the amount of the urine leaked, gender, activities, etc. They are usually single use only, which is important for hygiene, but for some people it is easier to wash the pads, and those people are provided with pads that can be used multiple times. Some products have chemical substances that, when in contact with urine, turn it into gel, change its colour (but not necessarily) and provide smell neutralization.

The type of incontinence influences the choice of *pads*. Some pads are more absorbent and used for moderate to severe incontinence, and some are smaller and used for smaller leakages. Some people have a problem with frequent urination of small amounts so, for them, some product in between is more suitable. Some people complain of incontinence-continence intervals that last for days. For better hygiene, it is better to change pads frequently, depending on the instructions of the manufacturer. Body-worn products can be in the form of *inserts* or *diapers*. Inserts are pads that are inserted into the underwear; they vary in size, thickness, and absorptive capacity. They have glue or another adhesive layer to fix the insert to the underwear. Diapers are products that can be single use only and disposable, or washable. They substitute for underwear and absorb the liquid. They are mostly used in people who have assistance with limited mobility. They can be either changed more frequently in people with severe incontinence condition or less frequently when leakage is only occasional.

Pull-ups and *pouches* are also in this group of products. Pull-ups are used as a replacement for underwear and can be either disposable or reusable. They look similar to diapers, except diapers are used when a person is being completely taken care of by another person, so they are designed for easy positioning and removal. Pull-up pants a person uses independently. They are indicated for moderate incontinence. For men, pads are not so comfortable, so they use them less frequently. For them, different absorptive products have been developed. They are called pouches, shields, or guards. They are designed to fit around the penis and scrotum, with special adaptations to hold them in place.

Underpads are towel- or blanket-like absorptive surfaces with outer hydrophobic, plastic material; they are placed under the person where he/she sits or lays. They are used for furniture protection and are indicated for people who have trouble with night urination and incontinence as well, or whenever there is a chance for urine leakage and contamination of furniture. Skin protection and care are here important, especially if the person has low immunity and is prone to infections.

These products, no matter which size, have hydrophilic and hydrophobic component. Hydrophilic means absorptive and its thickness determines the frequency of changing or washing it. The hydrophobic component ensures that there is no wetting of the clothes or surroundings. Skin care is essential, because skin can be irritated because of the occlusion and contact with synthetic materials.

9.2 Sheaths and bags

Sheaths are also called external catheters, condom catheters, or uridoms. They are used by men who have moderate to severe incontinence. A sheath is a penile cover that is connected to a bag. Both are made of synthetic materials such as latex, silicone, or rubber. A health care provider should educate men how to use this product, emphasizing that it is important to keep the skin dry, clean, and not irritated. Some men are allergic to latex, and that should be kept in mind, before deciding to use it. Sheaths are indicated in men who are independent, but have limited mobility, or are in wheelchairs; they should be able to change the bag and sheath by themselves. It is not recommended for people with loss of memory or neural damage to sensations of the pelvis. Some men who do not want to use pads, or are unsatisfied with them, can use sheaths, and it has been shown to preserve their dignity and style. The placement of the sheath is simple but a man should first pick the right size of the product and determine whether he is allergic either to latex or the adhesive inside the sheath. The adhesive is active when it is slightly warmed up. The sheath is connected to a bag. Before putting on a new sheath, the skin must be properly washed with soap and water. Men who have or have had problems with infection are not good candidates for the sheath, since the product can stay in position for 24 hours or longer, which is a risk for infection, especially in immunocompromised older men.

However, the product is designed so that leakage is impossible, if properly placed. The size of the sheath is important and men should analyze manufacturers' instructions. If a sheath is compressing the penis, it could lead to swelling, damage to the skin, lack of blood circulation, and collection of venous blood. Even when the size is right, the glans shouldn't be compressed, so a gap should be left at the end of the sheath; however, that gap shouldn't be too large because it could induce bending of the tube and flow obstruction. Correct positioning is probably best done with the doctor's advice. The drainage bag is either detached in the underwear (for men in wheelchairs) or attached with an adhesive pad on the medial side of the thigh. Disposing of the bag content is in usual household conditions or as the manufacturer states in instructions. The product is protected from sudden rise in pressure under the speed of flow, and it won't rupture.

Collecting bags are attached to sheaths or indwelling catheters. Bags can be small for collecting small amounts of urine and bigger for night use. As previously said, a bag can be carried along attached on the inner side of the thigh or abdomen. For men who work or are outside for hours, this is a comfortable way of dealing with incontinence. Bags should be designed to fit with the clothes so they are not easily visible. Rarely, a side effect called purple urine bag syndrome can develop, for unknown reasons, and it is the cause of an intolerable smell. It is perhaps because of an interaction between the alkaline urine and gram-negative bacteria that produces purple pigment. This can be an indicator of an infection. When using these products, a person needs to be well educated and competent to clean in a proper way and, while doing so, to wear disposable gloves and to dispose of items in the right place. Before connecting to a new product, the skin needs to be washed and dried, and any irritation or symptoms of infection should be a sign not to put the product on, but rather to treat with creams and antibiotics.

9.3 Mechanical devices for incontinence

9.3.1 Female mechanical devices

Mechanical devices for women are called occlusive devices and their aim is to support the bladder neck, especially when a woman laughs, coughs, or strains. These products can be applied intraurethrally, externally over the opening of the urethra, or vaginally. The mechanism is the same: compression of the urethra and reducing the leakage.

External urethral devices use adhesive or mild suction to stay positioned on the outer opening of the female urethra. These products are not available in all markets, and their effectiveness has yet to be analyzed. The device is put over the opening of the urethra to block leaking or it compresses the distal urethra for a maximum of four hours or until voiding. Before voiding, the product is pulled out and washed, to be used again. Even though the studies have shown that 50% of people improved their condition, some people's incontinence worsened.

Intraurethral devices are usually used for training or other types of increased physical activity. Women with stress incontinence provoke their incontinence with intense physical activity, but mild physical activity can actually be helpful. These products are silicone cylinders that are inserted into the urethra, like plugs, and they have inner and outer parts that hold the product in place. The outer device is a retainer that keeps the product in the urethra and not the bladder, and holds onto the outer genitalia; the inner part is a balloon, inflated in the bladder, that provides occlusion and fixation from the proximal side and it is filled with air after insertion. The product is intended for temporary use and, if not used correctly, it can lead to complications. The intraurethral device is inserted with transducer or insertion probe. It is a small silicone tube with mineral oil and an insertion probe. As the product is being inserted, the liquid goes slowly from the proximal part to distal, which allows the product to pass though the urethra; but then it goes slowly back to the proximal part assuring the position with the balloon. They are intended for single use only, because they bring a high risk of infection. Some women complain of discomfort but, for others, after a few uncomfortable uses, they got used to having them in the urethra. This product is expensive when considering how often it should be changed. Because of the mechanical invasion on the urethral layer during placement/removal, some experience blood in urine.

Intravaginal devices can be tampons, pessaries, or contraceptive diaphragms. These are however, traditional forms of intravaginal devices that can be used for stress incontinence, but are actually produced for contraception. Other products that are specifically designed to treat stress incontinence are made of polyurethane or silicon. Their main purpose in stress incontinence is to support the bladder neck and prevent leaking with compression of urethra.

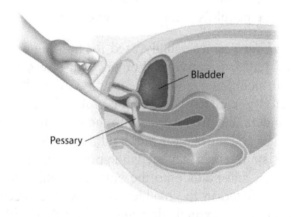

© Alila Medical Media - www.AlilaMedicalMedia.com

Figure 7 Installing of intravaginal pessary; occlusion of the urethra

The first group of products is designed as a removable, reusable ring made of silicone and it is difficult for some women to insert, especially if they have had vaginal surgeries. However, according to studies, women find it comfortable to wear and report that it improved their condition. The other product is made of polyurethane foam, is for single use, and is disposable. It is folded, but in contact with liquid it spreads and creates the occlusion. These devices are constructed for mild to moderate incontinence and showed good results in studies. However, some side effects have been reported: pain, infection, irritations, bleeding, urinary tract infection, and the lack of total continence.

9.3.2 Male mechanical devices

Male mechanical devices work by compressing the penis. There are two types of devices: a penile clamp and a peripenile strap. These devices are carefully placed, taking into account the circulation and skin integrity. Studies do not support the use of this product, so they are to be saved as the last resort.

The clamp consists of two attached parts that are covered on the inner side with sponge. That side goes in direct contact with the skin. Closing the clamp can be done with a ratchet system. Men who can use this product need to remember to remove it two hours after placement. The devices are recommended only for temporary use, during some intense physical activities that may induce incontinence.

9.4 Body-warn urinals

Female body-worn urinals are less successful in providing good adhesion, prevention of leakage, and good aesthetic results, than similar devices for the male. There are some products for women, but studies show that there are far better alternatives. The system includes a funnel-like part that guides the urine into a bag positioned between the legs, with or without attachments. Because of obvious anatomic differences, this kind of product gives a better result for males. *Male body-*

worn urinals (Dribble containers) are similar to sheaths, but some of the parts here are disposable and some are reusable. It is a plastic funnel-like sac for the penis and scrotum and it is attached on the other end to a disposable bag. Belts and straps are used to attach and position it. These products are recommended for men who didn't have success using pads or sheaths. The reason for that may be a retracted penis in elderly men. Here, also, it is important to take care of the hygiene and antibacterial environment.

9.5 Handheld urinals

Handheld urinal products are used for collecting urine when a person isn't able to access the toilet to empty the bladder because of immobility (severe arthritis, broken bones, or general weakness) or urge incontinence, when a person is outside the house and a toilet isn't always available, but the urge is strong. When this is the case, a person can't make it to a toilet in time, or isn't able to move, so they need a portable product to collect the urine. This product must be appropriate to gender, easy to use in bed or beside the bed where person lies or in a chair or wheelchair, but it requires assistance with emptying the urinal. The products are usually made of plastic, have various shapes and sizes that depend on the posture while voiding and body measures, but usually they are small so that they can be used in the car, for example, and they have a handle and are marked and graduated.

Female handheld urinals are appropriate for the female anatomy. The person using it must position the urinal under her and let the urine flow down. Depending on whether the urinal is properly held, and whether the woman's position is accurate (with legs a little apart), urine may or may not be spilled. That is why scientists have worked on a device that included a pump for emptying the urinal in a disposal container. The best position to urinate is to sit on the edge of the chair or bed, or stand. Women have more difficulties positioning the urinal correctly to prevent spilling. That is why there are various sizes and shapes on the market, so the user can find the adequate one.

Male handheld urinals include a tube-like part for insertion of the penis, and they are therefore easier to use. Some of the products have a valve that prevents the spilling. The product may be attached to a container.

The use of urinals sometimes requires some assistance from other people. Also, it is useful for a person to have suitable clothes that can be easily removed to facilitate urination without staining. The products are usually made reusable and they are cleaned with water and soap. Some devices are fit to be used in hospitals, or at home or outside, and the latter can fit into a pocket, but there are also urinals that are made of cardboard and therefore for single use only and disposable.

9.6 Commodes and bedpans

Commodes and bedpans are made for elderly and immobile people. For them, there are various toilet adaptations, such as holders, raised toilet seats, and bidets, but in some cases a person can't get to the bathroom. Here, it is much safer and easier to use bedpans or commodes. They require a second person for assistance to get on the bedpan or commode safely. **Bedpans** have a similar purpose as portable urinals, but they are bigger and modified according to person's illness. For example, there are special bedpans for pelvic fractures and femur fractures. Bedpans are usually made of plastic, for easy cleaning, and can be sterilized in an autoclave in the nursing home. Bedpans require a person to sit in the bed and that can be especially difficult for elderly people and those with reduced mobility, lack of strength, obesity. A position on the side can be tried, but it requires protective sheaths and other objects to guide the urine in the bedpan. A person should have privacy, but not when there's a very high risk of falling, and then he/she shouldn't be alone. He/she shouldn't sit for long, because that could lead to pressure-induced injuries. Bedpans are recommended for use only by people who don't get out of bed at all. When it is difficult to position the person onto the bedpan, in most of the cases, commodes are used instead.

Commodes can be either shower chairs that are modified to be used as portable toilets, or they are reserved just for the latter function. A commode is shaped like a chair, can stand beside the bed, and has a container that is easily detached and emptied. However, the positioning of the person onto this toilet may be difficult for an assistant, depending on the person's weight and mobility. Then, after he/she sits, it is important to give them privacy, but also to make sure that they won't fall out of the toilet. There is a product called "three in one" that provides mobility, safety, and higher seat, which means less difficulty in moving from the bed or wheelchair to toilet. A product needs to fit the person (it is not safe for some obese people to use it); the handles must be reachable, reducing the risk of falling; it must be comfortable, so some pads or pillows can be attached; aesthetics are important (it needs to be covered to not look like a toilet), and it should have foot supports, since a user may sit on it for a while, and the legs are in better position. The use of commodes requires some assistance from other people, either health care providers or family members. Usually, the problem is with cleaning. For that reason, and for the sake of sterilization, better care for hygiene, and maintaining antibacterial surroundings, it is usually best for the person to be taken care of by a professional.

9.7 Indwelling catheters

Catheterisation is a method of inserting a tube-catheter in a sterile environment to empty the bladder. Female catheters are about 25cm long and male catheters are 40-45cm long. The size is measured in Frenches, and they range from 8 to 26 F. The catheter drain the urine into a bag, which may be attached to the skin. Intermittent catheterisation is indicated when retention of urine occurs. The catheter should be removed immediately when the bladder is emptied. Catheterisation and wearing the catheter bring some risks, since the procedure is invasive: urinary tract infection, injury, stone development, and other less frequent problems can occur. A catheter may be inserted for a longer period; then a special regimen is followed. Catheters can be *intraurethral* or *suprapubic*.

Intraurethral catheters are inserted into the urethra, which can be damaged from the inside during the insertion; that could be a good condition for bacterial invasion and infection, especially in people who are prone to infection (those with diabetes mellitus). This approach is usually used for intermittent catheterisation.

Suprapubic catheterisation is done through a small incision in the abdominal wall. Health care providers prefer this approach in long-term use of a catheter, since it doesn't damage the urethra, the catheter stays in place, and thus the genitals are left free of catheterisation. The disadvantages are that, shortly after the surgical procedure, people complain of hypersensitivity of the area, and sometimes bladder spasms can develop; there may be difficulty sitting, which is more likely with obese people, and discharge from the catheter site. When removing the suprapubic catheter, it is important to manipulate the catheter carefully, since tissue in the inner part may have developed a granulation around the catheter as a reaction to a foreign body.

The materials from which the catheters are made are silicone, silicone-elastomer coated latex, or hydrophilic polymer-coated latex. These materials cause the least friction and tissue reaction, are soft and comfortable, and form a barrier against bacteria. Catheters mustn't fall out of the bladder, but have to be easy to remove. They have a balloon that inflates when the catheter is inserted to secure its position. However, latex should be avoided because of possible allergies.

A catheterisation in some people can last for 3-5 years, or even up to 20 years in people with unmanageable problems. This is called indwelling catheterisation. Intermittent catheterisation (maximum 14 days) is used when a person undergoes surgery, when urine is monitored in the hospital, and to drain urine in acute or chronic retention. Indwelling catheters are changed and replaced in a maximum of seven days. Indications for long-term catheterisation are outflow obstructions, neurological conditions that cause chronic retention, and paralysis.

The most common complication of catheterisation, as previously stated, is urinary tract infection. The bacteria come from both the colon and the skin of the perineum, and travel to the site of the damaged epithelium, or they are transferred from the hands of a person taking care of the catheter site. Symptoms of urinary infection vary from no symptoms at all to dysuria, pain, itchiness during urination, blood in the urine, lumbar pain, fever, fatigue, and chills. Using this product, the growth of bacteria is imminent in four weeks after catheter placement, but a significant number of bacteria, which is 100,000, is a sign of infection. Even if catheterisation is a predisposing condition, prophylactic doses of antibiotics are not recommended, because the bacteria become resistant to them. The best practice is to use the urinoculture sample, do an antibiogram-sensitivity test for antibiotics, and treat the infection accordingly. Other complications include blood in urine, catheter blockages, urine leakage around the catheter, and the catheter pulling out of the correct position. If a person has blood in urine, it could be because of the recent catheterisation or a sign of infection or other injuries, in which case a health care professional needs to unblock the drainage. The catheter can be blocked when, after long-term use, calcium begins to precipitate. In this case, the catheter should be changed early. Catheters are changed depending on the condition, but on average every three months. Urine can leak when the catheter is blocked; in this case, also, the catheter should be removed. Other causes of leakage are bladder spasms that can be induced by either the presence of the catheter or the size of the balloon, which, if larger than it should be, compresses the walls and induces contractions.

The care of the catheter depends on the frequency with which it is changed, hygiene, disinfection and antibacterial environment, and on observing the condition of the urine and catheter: whether the colour of urine is yellow, its turbidity, existence of blockages, etc. [14] [76]

10. Complications of incontinence and effect on life

Skin problems - Irritation of the vulva may develop because of the wetness of the perineal area. Other than that, the skin is prone to rashes and infections. Irritation should be treated with adequate hygiene, washing with water and soap, and drying the skin. Neutralizing creams are used for calming down the skin. If incontinence products are used, adequate care is based on the manufacturers' instructions, but also requires hygiene and proper changing or washing of the products.

Unpleasant odours – are a common complaint of people, because of the accumulation of the urine and the possible contact with bacteria. These are hidden with pads incorporating chemicals that turn the liquid into gel and neutralize the smell. Here also the adequate degree of hygiene and changing of the pads is imperative.

Urinary tract infections (UTIs) and especially, repeated urinary infections, can easily develop, because of weakness of the sphincter and the fact that the pathway to the bladder is open for bacterial breach.

Working life is affected when the employee must take frequent breaks for bathroom visits and the productivity is thereby lowered. Also, a person's attention is divided by expectations of urine leakage, thoughts about how to postpone the micturation, and worry about the obviousness of the condition, including whether other colleagues are aware of how frequently the person goes to the bathroom, smells, and discomfort of the person in general. Also, if urine leaks when lifting heavy objects, a person may have to be repositioned to work at something else.

Personal life is affected on many levels. Lack of self-confidence and a sense of shame and embarrassment are present with many people. Some of them develop anxiety and depression because of thoughts of being exposed and stigmata from other people, the lack of motivation and self-respect, and resultant sadness. Social life is also affected because a person with this condition is more likely to start avoiding other people and public places, because of the social stigma and unavailability of toilets. That brings a sense of loneliness and helplessness. Relationship with a partner may be damaged or people may complain of tension, anxiety, pressure, lack of emotional support, or, in many cases, a person's fear of not having support, and then hiding the problem between them and their partners, which affects sex life.

11. Education, health promotion, and prevention

The primary aim of health care professionals should be *education*, primary prevention, and maintaining continence. Even though incontinence can be successfully treated, if the population were aware of the risks that promote incontinence and measures that can lessen the risks and *promote health*, they would behave accordingly to maintain continence as long as possible and have control over their health. With information widely spread among the population, awareness grows, and the social stigma is less.

First, it is important to spread the information about why incontinence happens, what the risks are, and how it is treatable. If the family knows about the nature of this illness, then individual family support is higher. Family support is the basis for treatment and prevention, since it encourages and motivates the person. With more information, a person who has a problem with incontinence will more likely seek help; at least, that is the goal. This information is provided through posters, Internet articles, pamphlets, lectures, seminars, printed self-care instructions, and activities of health care professionals. The sources of information may or may not be reliable and the job of a health care professional should be to guide people to sources of correct information. Some studies showed that people wait a year before seeking help and other studies showed that they wait between 2 and 11 years; during that period, they cope with the condition in their own ways, increasing the risk of complications and decreasing their quality of life. [77] [78] Some people report that they thought the problem was transient, or that they would manage it by themselves, or that they were embarrassed to admit to the health care professional that there was a problem. On the other hand, an HCP is responsible for the general health of his patient and not just for the problem that they admitted having. If an HCP offers a conversation about any problem that bothers his patient, he or she, in confidence, may speak up about the problem. The HCP should also be aware of the measures that a person should perform in order to prevent or treat the condition. Some people reported that their family doctor assured them that it is a normal advent that comes with aging, which is not entirely true. Since those most likely to be affected are women and the elderly, prevention and education is directed towards these two groups. Target issues are risk factors and management. All health care professionals need to be well informed and able to provide the patients with correct answers. Good communication between the HCP and the rest of the population is crucial. It is important not to raise expectations beyond the possible. Each person should be able to easily get other people's experiences as their own motivation. That is why some speakers about incontinence may invite patients to speak up about their problems, if they are willing. There are organisations to which a person with bladder problem can go or look into to be more informed.

A person's correct actions to solve the problem are not the only important factors. It is also important for doctors to recognize the risks in certain groups of people. Pregnant women should know that, with pregnancy, the pelvic floor muscles can be weakened, which could lead to a few problems. In time, they can start practicing Kegel exercises to strengthen the pelvic floor.

Prevention is primary (modifying the risk factors before the illness develops), secondary (screening and treatment of the targeted population), tertiary (treating the illness and preventing further damage and complications). Primary prevention lies in educating the population and depends on the knowledge provided. Primary prevention is the task not only of primary care physicians and nurses, but also of family members and loved ones. Modifying risk factors include smoking cessation, dieting, mild physical activity, and maintaining a healthy weight.

Reduction of smoking is confirmed by some studies to have a beneficial effect on incontinence. Smoking induces coughing, which provokes the incontinence by creating high abdominal pressure, affecting the pelvic floor.

Eating healthy is also important because eating dry, fast food that lacks fibre can lead to constipation and stool impaction, which then compresses the bladder and stimulates the contractions and incontinence. Losing sufficient weight is recommended, since it can decrease the number of incontinence episodes. Habits in drinking and going to the bathroom can also be organised differently. A person should drink 2 litres of water a day in normal conditions. That requires frequent bathroom visits. But it is not recommended to go to the bathroom before the need to empty the bladder occurs. A person shouldn't drink less than 2 litres, because that brings other problems, such as infections and dehydration. On the other hand, drinking too much water worsens the incontinence for obvious reason (more urine is produced). Caffeine and alcohol should be reduced. Caffeine acts like a diuretic and alcohol can affect incontinence acutely and chronically. Alcohol induces voiding and causes sedation.

Kegel exercises and other exercises of the pelvic floor can be very useful in men, as well as in women. Doing exercises correctly and regularly can help to prevent incontinence, and the treatment methods bring better results.

Secondary and tertiary approached have been previously covered. Adequate, on-time treatment reduces problems with micturation and improves the quality of life. [14]

Works Cited

1. **Barron, J.** The Physiology of the Urinary System. *Baseline of health foundation.* [Online] [Cited: 10 07, 2016.] https://jonbarron.org/article/physiology-urinary-system.

2. *The role of pelvic organs prolapse in the etiology of urinary incontinence in women.* **Zargham M, Alizadeh F, Moayednia A, Haghdani S, Nouri-Mahdavi K.** 2013, Adv Biomed Res, p. 6.2:22.

3. Five Facts about XX or XY. *Gender selection authority.* [Online] 10 07, 2016. https://www.genderselectionauthority.com/blog/five-facts-about-xx-or-xy.

4. Difference Between Male and Female Urinary System. *TheyDiffer.com.* [Online] [Cited: 10 07, 2016.] http://theydiffer.com/difference-between-male-and-female-urinary-system/.

5. *Management of overactive bladder and urge urinary incontinence in the elderly patient.* **Erdem N, Chu FM.** 2006, Am J Med, pp. 119(3 Suppl 1):29-36.

6. *Clinical practice. Urinary stress incontinence in women.* **RG, Rogers.** March 6, 2008, N Engl J Med, pp. 358(10):1029-36.

7. **Vasavada SP.** Urinary Incontinence. *Medscape.* [Online] 10 27, 2015. [Cited: 10 12, 2016.] http://emedicine.medscape.com/article/452289-overview.

8. **Liedl, B, Schorsch, I ,Stief, C.** The development of concepts of female (in)continence. Pathophysiology, diagnostics and surgical therapy. *Urologe A(44)Nr7.* 2005.

9. Urge Incontinence. *WebMED.* [Online] 04 23, 2016. [Cited: 10 08, 2016.] http://www.webmd.com/urinary-incontinence-oab/america-asks-11/urge.

10. Overflow Incontinence. *WebMED.* [Online] [Cited: 10 08, 2016.] http://www.webmd.com/urinary-incontinence-oab/overflow-incontinence.

11. Functional Incontinence. *WebMED.* [Online] [Cited: 10 08, 2016.] http://www.webmd.com/urinary-incontinence-oab/functional-incontinence.

12. Mixed Incontinence. *WebMED.* [Online] [Cited: 10 08, 2016.] http://www.webmd.com/urinary-incontinence-oab/mixed-incontinence.

13. *Prevalence of urinary incontinence in men, women, and children—current evidence: findings of the Fourth International Consultation on Incontinence.* **Buckley BS, Lapitan MCM.** 2010, Urology, pp. 76(2):265–70.

14. **Paul Abrams, Linda Cardozo, Saad Khoury, Alan Wein.** *Incontinence.* 5th. Ohio Valley Goodwill Cincinnati (Cincinnati, OH, U.S.A.) : Health Publications Ltd, 2013.

15. *The prevalence of urinary incontinence 20 years after childbirth: a national cohort study in singleton primiparae after vaginal or caesarean delivery.* **Gyhagen M, Bullarbo M, Nielsen TF, et al.** 2013, BJOG, pp. 120(2):144-51.

16. *Prevalence and risk factors for urinary and fecal incontinence four months after vaginal delivery.* **Baydock SA, Flood C,**

Schulz JA, et al; . 2009 Jan, J Obstet Gynaecol Can, pp. 31(1):36-41.

17. *Risk factors for urinary, fecal, or dual incontinence in the Nurses' Health Study.* **Matthews CA, Whitehead WE, Townsend MK, et al.** 2013, Obstet Gynecol, pp. 122(3):539-45.

18. *Exclusive caesarean section delivery and subsequent urinary and faecal incontinence: a 12-year longitudinal study.* **MacArthur C, Glazener C, Lancashire R, et al.** 2011, BJOG, pp. 118(8):1001-7.

19. *Vaginal hysterectomy and risk of pelvic organ prolapse and stress urinary incontinence surgery.* **Forsgren C, Lundholm C, Johansson AL, et al.** 2012, Int Urogynecol J, pp. 23(1):43-8.

20. *Menopausal transition and the risk of urinary incontinence: results from a British prospective cohort.* **Mishra GD, Cardozo L, Kuh D.** 2010, BJU Int, pp. 106(8):1170-5.

21. Urinary incontinence in neurological disease: assessment and management. *NICE National Institute for Heath and Care Excellence.* [Online] August 2012. [Cited: 10 12, 2016.] https://www.nice.org.uk/guidance/cg148/chapter/introduction.

22. *Body mass index, weight gain, and incident urinary incontinence in middle-aged women.* **Townsend MK, Danforth KN, Rosner B, et al.** 2007, Obstet Gynecol, pp. 110(2 Pt 1):346-53.

23. *Parity is not associated with urgency with or without urinary incontinence.* **Hirsch AG, Minassian VA, Dilley A, et al.** 2010, Int Urogynecol J, pp. 21(9):1095-102.

24. *Urinary incontinence in women, without manifest injury to the bladder 1914.* **Kelly HA, Dumm WM.** 1998, Int Urogynecol J Pelvic Floor Dysfunct, pp. 9(3):158-64.

25. *On diurnal incontinence of urine in women.* **V., Bonney.** 1923, J Obstet Gynaecol Br Emp, pp. 30:358–365.

26. *A method for evaluating the stress of urinary incontinence.* **Barnes, A.** 1940, Am J Obstet Gynecol, pp. 40:381–90.

27. *Urethral closure studied with cineroentgenography and simultaneous bladder-urethra pressure recording.* **Enhornung G, Miller ER, Hinman F Jr.** Mar 1964, Surg Gynecol Obstet, pp. 118:507-16.

28. *Stress urinary incontinence.* **McGuire EJ, Lytton B, Pepe V, Kohorn EI.** 1976, Obstet Gynecol, pp. 47:255–264.

29. **Green TH, Jr.** 1968, Obstet Gynecol SurveyClassification of stress urinary incontinence in the female: an appraisal of its current status, pp. 23:632–634.

30. *Stress urinary incontinence: where are we now, where should we go?* **DeLancey, JO.** 1996, Am J Obstet Gynecol, pp. 175:311–319.

31. *An integral theory of female urinary incontinence: experimental and clinical considerations.* **Petros PE, Ulmsten UI.** 1990, Acta Obstet Gynecol Scand Suppl., pp. 153:7–31.

32. *Urethral pressure and power generation during coughing and voluntary contraction of the pelvic floor in females with genuine stress incontinence.* **G, Lose.** 1991, Br J Urol, pp. 67:580–585.

33. *Anatomical and physiological observations on the supraspinal control of bladder and urethral sphincter muscles in*

the cat. **Holstege G, Griffiths D, de Wall H, Dalm E.** 1986, J Comp Neurol, pp. 250:449–61.

34. *Urinary Tract Infection and Neurogenic Bladder.* **McKibben MJ, Seed P, Ross SS, Borawski KM.** 2015, Urol Clin North Am, pp. 42(4):527-36.

35. *The aging bladder: morphology and urodynamics.* **Elbadawi A, Diokno A, Millard R.** 1998, World J Urol , pp. 16(suppl 1):S10-S34.

36. *Estrogen Treatment for Urinary Incontinence: Never, Now, or in the Future?* **DuBeau, CE.** 2005, JAMA, pp. 293:998–1001.

37. *Is Estrogen for Urinary Incontinence Good or Bad?* **Dae Kyung Kim, Michael B Chancellor.** 2006, Rev Urol, pp. 8(2): 91–92.

38. *Levator ani muscle stretch induced by simulated vaginal birth.* **Lien, KC, et al.** 2004, Obstet Gynecol, pp. 103(1):p.31-40.

39. *Urinary incontinence after vaginal delivery or cesarean section.* **Rortveit G, Daltveit AK, Hannestad YS, Hunskaar S, Norwegian ES.** 2003, N Engl J Med , pp. 348:900-7.

40. *Anal function: effect of pregnancy and delivery.* **Chaliha C, Sultan AH, Bland JM, Monga AK, Stanton SL.** 2001 Aug, Am J Obstet Gynecol, pp. 185(2):427-32.

41. *Factors that are associated with clinically overt postpartum urinary retention after vaginal delivery.* **Carley ME, Carley JM, Vasdev G, et al.** 2002, Am Jo of Obs and Gyn , pp. 187: 430-433.

42. *Diagnostic evaluation of urinary incontinence in geriatric patients.* **BD, Weiss.** 1998, Am Fam Physician, pp. 57(11):2675–84.

43. *The role of the primary care physician in the management of bladder dysfunction.* **Imam, KA.** 2004, Rev Urol., pp. 6(suppl 1):S38–S44.

44. **Albo M, Richter HE.** Urodynamic testing. [Online] Feb 2014. [Cited: 10 10, 2016.] https://www.niddk.nih.gov/health-information/health-topics/diagnostic-tests/urodynamic-testing/Pages/Urodynamic%20Testing.aspx.

45. Urinary incontinence. *Mayo clinic.* [Online] [Cited: 10 09, 2016.] http://www.mayoclinic.org/diseases-conditions/urinary-incontinence/basics/symptoms/con-20037883.

46. *Self-efficacy mechanisms in human agency.* **A, Bandura.** s.l. : American Psychologist, 1982, pp. 37:122–147.

47. *The impact of female urinary incontinence and urgency on quality of life and partner relationship.* **Nilsson M, Lalos A, Lalos O.** 2009, Neurol Urodyn, pp. 28:976–81.

48. *Too wet to exercise? Leaking urine as a barrier to physical activity in women.* **Brown WJ, MillerYD.** 2001, J Sci Med Sport, pp. 4:373–8.

49. *Review The psychosocial impact of urinary incontinence in women.* **Sinclair AJ, Ramsay IN.** 2011, The Obstetrician & Gynaecologist, pp. 13:143–148.

50. *A review of the psychosocial predictors of help seeking behaviour and impact on quality of life in people with urinary incontinence.* **C., Shaw.** 2001, J Clin Nurs, pp. 10:15–24.

51. *A new questionnaire for urinary incontinence diagnosis in women: development and testing.* **Bradley CS, Rovner ES, Morgan MA, Berlin M, Novi JM, Shea JA, Arya LA.** January 2005 , Am J Obstet Gynecol, pp. 192(1):66-73.

52. Pelvic exam. *MAYO clinic.* [Online] May 09, 2014. [Cited: 10 10, 2016.] http://www.mayoclinic.org/tests-procedures/pelvic-exam/basics/what-you-can-expect/prc-20013064.

53. Bladder stress test and bonney test for urinary incontinence in women. *Healthwise.* [Online] Sept 09, 2014. [Cited: Oct 10, 2016.] http://www.webmd.com/urinary-incontinence-oab/bladder-stress-test-and-bonney-test-for-urinary-incontinence-in-women.

54. Q test. *Urinary incontinence in adults.* [Online] [Cited: October 10, 2016.] http://www.ouhsc.edu/geriatricmedicine/education/incontinence/INCONTQTip_Test.htm.

55. **Manski D.** Stress Urinary Incontinence in Women (2/3). *www.urology-textbook.com.* [Online] [Cited: 10 10, 2016.] http://www.urology-textbook.com/stress-urinary-incontinence-diagnosis.html.

56. Diagnosing urinary incontinence. *NHS choices.* [Online] 10 06, 2016. [Cited: 10 15, 2016.] http://www.nhs.uk/Conditions/Incontinence-urinary/Pages/Diagnosis.aspx.

57. Michigan Healthy Healing After Delivery Program / Urogynecology. *University of Michigean health system.* [Online] [Cited: 10 12, 2016.] http://careguides.med.umich.edu/post-void-residual-pvr-test.

58. *Measurement of postvoid residual urine with portable transabdominal bladder ultrasound scanner and urethral*

catheterization. **Goode PS, Locher JL, Bryant RL, Roth DL, Burgio KL.** 2000, Int Urogynecol J Pelvic Floor Dysfunct, pp. 11:296-300.

59. **Blaivas J, Chancellor MB, Weiss J, Verhaaren M.** *Atlas of urodynamics.* Malden,USA : Blackwell Publishing, 2007.

60. *Is urethral pressure profilometry a useful diagnostic test for stress urinary incontinence?* **AM, Weber.** 2001 Nov, Obstet Gynecol Surv, pp. 56(11):720-35.

61. *Bulbocavernous reflex revisited.* **Vodusek, DB.** 2003, Neurourology & Urodynamics, pp. 22,681–682.

62. **Ince, Susan.** Better Bladder and Bowel Control. *Harvard Medical School.* [Online] [Cited: 10 13, 2016.] http://www.patienteducationcenter.org/articles/better-bladder-and-bowel-control/.

63. *Expanded indications for the pubovaginal sling: treatment of type 2 or 3 stress incontinence.* **MR, Zaragoza.** Nov 1996, J Urol, pp. 156(5):1620-2.

64. **Gill BC, Rackley RR, Firoozi F.** Injectable Bulking Agents for Incontinence. *Medscape.* [Online] [Cited: 10 15, 2016.] http://emedicine.medscape.com/article/447068-overview#a4.

65. **Molden SM, Lucente VR, Mastropietro MA.** Suburethral sling procedures. *Glowm.* [Online] 2016. [Cited: 10 15, 2016.] http://www.glowm.com/section_view/heading/Suburethral%20Sling%20Procedures/item/68.

66. **Vasavada SP, Rackley R,.** Vaginal Sling Procedures. *Med scape .* [Online] 2015. [Cited: 10 15, 2016.] http://emedicine.medscape.com/article/447951-overview#a3.

67. *Burch colposuspension versus fascial sling to reduce urinary stress incontinence.* **Albo ME, Richter HE, Brubaker L, et al.** May 24, 2007 , N Engl J Med, pp. 356(21):2143-55.

68. **Siff L,Ellsworth PI, Ferzandi TR.** Burch Colposuspension. *Medscape.* [Online] [Cited: 10 17, 2016.] http://emedicine.medscape.com/article/1893728-overview#a3.

69. **Sajadi KP, Terris MK,.** Artificial Urinary Sphincter Placement Treatment & Management. *Medscape.* [Online] [Cited: 10 15, 2016.] http://emedicine.medscape.com/article/443737-treatment#d10.

70. **Ellsworth, PI.** Sacral Nerve Stimulation. *Medscape.* [Online] 12 09, 2015. [Cited: 10 17, 2016.] http://emedicine.medscape.com/article/2036909-overview.

71. *Percutaneous Tibial Nerve Stimulation: A Clinically and Cost Effective Addition to the Overactive Bladder Algorithm of Care.* **Staskin, D R, Peters, KM, MacDiarmid, S, Shore, N, de Groat, W.C.** 2012, Current Urology Reports, pp. 327–34.

72. **Wooldridge, LS.** About Incontinence - Treatment/Management Options - Percutaneous Tibial Nerve Stimulation (PTNS). *The Simon Foundation for Continence.* [Online] 02 26, 2016. [Cited: 10 17, 2016.] http://www.simonfoundation.org/About_Incontinence_Treatment_Options_Percutaneous_Tibial_Nerve_Stimulation.html.

73. **Ellsworth PI, Kim ED.** Botulinum Toxin Injections for Neurogenic Detrusor Overactivity Technique. *Medscape.* [Online] 01 13, 2016. [Cited: 10 17, 2016.] http://emedicine.medscape.com/article/2036931-technique.

74. *European experience of 200 cases treated with botulinum-A toxin injections into the detrusor muscle for urinary incontinence*

due to neurogenic detrusor overactivity. **Reitz A, Stöhrer M, Kramer G, Del Popolo G, Chartier-Kastler E, Pannek J, Burgdörfer H, Göcking K, Madersbacher H, Schumacher S, Richter R, von Tobel J, Schurch B.** April 2004, Eur Urol, pp. 45(4):510-5.

75. *Botulinum toxin injections for adults with overactive bladder syndrome.* **Duthie JB, Vincent M, Herbison GP, Wilson DI, Wilson D.** Dec 2011, Cochrane Database Syst Rev, p. (12):CD005493.

76. *Continence Product Advisor.* [Online] International Consultation on Incontinence, International Continence Society. [Cited: 10 15, 2016.] http://www.continenceproductadvisor.org/Products.

77. *Factors associated with women's decisions to seek treatment for urinary incontinence.* **Kinchen KS, Burgio K, Diokno AC, Fultz NH, Bump R,Obenchain R.** 2003, J WomensHealth (Larchmt), pp. 12:687-98.

78. *Characteristics of female outpatients with urinary incontinence participating in a 6-month observational study in 14 European countries. .* **Sykes D, R. Castro, et al.** 2005, Maturitas, pp. 52:S13-S23.

79. *Urodynamic Studies in Adults: AUA/SUFU Guideline.* **Winters JC, Dmochowski RR, Goldman HB, Herndon CDA, Kobashi KC, Kraus SR, et al.** 2012, J Urol, pp. 188(6):2455-63.